Eucalyptus

HUNDREDS OF
HOUSEHOLD USES

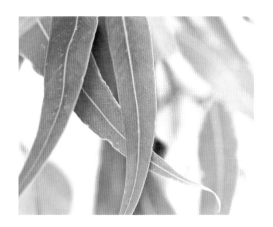

Publisher's Note:
All reasonable care has been exercised by the author and publisher to ensure that the tips and remedies included in this guide are simple and safe. However, it is important to note that all uses of eucalyptus should be practised with caution and a doctor's, or relevant professional's, advice should be sought if in any doubt or before any topical or medicinal usage – the advice in this book is not a replacement for that of a doctor. The author, editors and publisher take no responsibility for any consequences of any application which results from reading the information contained herein.

A note on measurements:
Please note also that the measurements provided in this book are presented as metric/imperial/US-cups practical equivalents, and that all eggs are medium (UK)/large (US) respectively unless otherwise stated.

This is a **FLAME TREE** book
First published in 2012

Publisher and Creative Director: Nick Wells
Project Editor: Laura Bulbeck
Picture Research: Lydia Good and Laura Bulbeck
Art Director: Mike Spender
Layout Design: Dave Jones
Digital Design and Production: Chris Herbert
Proofreader: Alex Davidson
Indexer: Helen Snaith

Special thanks to Jane Ashley.

14 16 15 13

3 5 7 9 10 8 6 4

FLAME TREE PUBLISHING
Crabtree Hall, Crabtree Lane
Fulham, London SW6 6TY
United Kingdom

www.flametreepublishing.com

© 2012 Flame Tree Publishing Ltd

ISBN 978-0-85775-618-3

A CIP Record for this book is available from the British Library upon request.

Every effort has been made to contact copyright holders. We apologise in advance for any omissions and would be pleased to insert the appropriate acknowledgement in subsequent editions of this publication.

Printed in China

The following images are courtesy of **Shutterstock** and © the following contributors:
1, 158b, 168, 169, 175t, 175b Richard Griffin; 5l & 91 Gtranquillity; 5r & 66r Margaret M Stewart; 6 Kaspars Grinvalds; 7 Layland Masuda; 8, 75, 112, 121 Africa Studio; 9 Tikona; 11 Robyn Mackenzie; 13 RobynButler; 14b JanelleLugge; 14t MelBrackstone; 15 Yuttasak Jannarong; 26 SteveLovegrove; 32 Salim October; 33 markrhiggins; 35l Deamer; 36 edella; 37 LouLouPhotos; 38 Blackpixel; 39 Sergey Mironov; 41, 141 Sandra Cunningham; 43, 113, 136, 139 Piotr Marcinski; 44 Gunnar Pippel; 45 Thinglass; 46 Norman Pogson; 47 djem; 48 Candace Hartley; 49 BW Folsom; 51l, 100 Goodluz; 51r Peter zijlstra; 53, 105 matka_Wariatka; 55, 78l lightpoet; 56t Elena Elisseeva; 56b Photoroller; 57 WouterTolenaars; 58 Janis Smits; 59 OlivierLe Queinec; 60r jocic; 60l karam Miri; 61 Iwona Grodzka; 62 Jozef of Szara Fabiani; 63 Iriana Shiyan; 65 Paul Matthew Photography; 66l Joe Gough; 67l Galushko Sergey; 67l Neftali; 69 Matthew Collingwood; 70b, 150t Daniel Krylov; 70t Graça Victoria; 71 Balazs Justin; 72l, 103 wavebreakmediaLtd; 72r Ctatiana; 73b cheyennezj; 73t ester22; 76t, 132 MonkeyBusiness Images; 76b Hywit Dimyadi; 77 Lein deLeon; 78r PeJo; 79r OlivierLe Moal; 79l SinisaBotas; 81 AnetaPics; 82 & 86b NikolaiTsvetkov; 84 Francesco Scotto; 84 VitalyTitov & Maria Sidelnikova; 85 MelissaBouyounan; 86t sixninepixels; 87 XAOC; 88 Annette Shaff; 89t AlexKalashnikov; 89b, 134 Lusoimages; 93, 167 Subbotina Anna; 94 prodakszyn; 96, 135 discpicture; 97b Julija Sapic; 97t Lasse Kristensen; 98 Sukharevskyy Dmytro (nevodka); 99 & 104 hsagencia; 101 Noam Armonn; 102 sheff; 106t Diego Cervo; 106b g215; 107 Tandem; 108 Shane White; 109 Imcsike; 110, 116 Richard MLee; 111 ponsulak kunsub; 114 Route66; 117 Fedulova Olga; 118 Dmitriy Shironosov; 119 pukach; 120, 129 Lenetstan; 122 deepblue-photographer; 123 andreasnikolas; 124 Arman Zhenikeyev; 125 vupulepe; 126 decathlon; 127l Christo; 127r sai0112; 128 Katia Vasileva; 130 Robert Kneschke; 131 Andresr; 137 Sheldunov Andrew; 138t negativkz; 138b Rasulov; 143 Kurhan; 144 Ron Zmiri; 145 Celso Diniz; 146t Brian Holm Nielsen; 146b ScottLatham; 147 BrandonBlinkenberg; 149t palex1977; 149b picsbyst; 150b Jeka; 151 Stocksnapper; 153 Gyuszkofoto; 155 DarrenBaker; 156b Madlen; 156t NinaMalyna; 157 T-Design; 158t TimothyLarge; 159 sevenke; 160b AnnaIA; 160t & 180 Tompet; 161 Tyler Olson; 162 joingate; 163 Rtimages; 164 Arpi; 165 DenisNata; 170 c.byatt norman; 171 Kirk Peart Professional Imaging; 172 mikeledray; 173 Coprid; 174 ChristinaRichards; 176 Arvydas Kniuksta; 177 Petrov Anton; 178 David Hyde; 179 Dervin Witmer; 181 Arkady; 182 Dirk Ott; 183 AlexanderRaths; 185 Shcherbakov Ilya; 186r Cosmin Manci; 186l ZoomTeam; 187 Aaron Amat; 188 mihalec; and courtesy of **Wikimedia Commons** (via the Creative Commons Attribution-Share Alike 3.0 Unported license and/or the Creative Commons Attribution-Share Alike 2.0/2.5 Generic license and/or the GNU Free Documentation License and/or public domain) and the following suppliers: 3 & 23 Wouter Hagens; 17, 22 Danielle Langlois; 18 Matilda; 19 Wittylama; 20t & 192, 25, 29 Melburnian; 20b Mike Bayly; 21 JJ Harrison (jjharrison89@facebook.com); 24 Daderot; 27 Stan Shebs; 28 amandabhslater; 30 Owheelj; 31 © Jean Tosti; 189 Forest & Kim Starr.

Eucalyptus

HUNDREDS OF
HOUSEHOLD USES

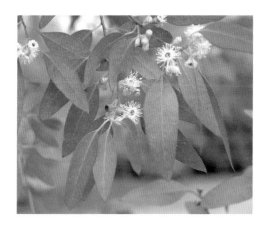

Lesley Dobson

**FLAME TREE
PUBLISHING**

Contents

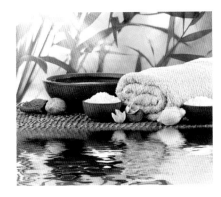
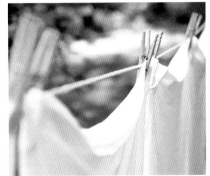

Introduction

There are around 750 species of eucalyptus, nearly all of which come originally from Australia (where they are a firm favourite of the koalas who live there), although some now grow in over 90 countries around the world. With the right consideration and care you could even grow a eucalyptus in your own garden or as a house plant that will brighten your home with its blossom's stunning colours.

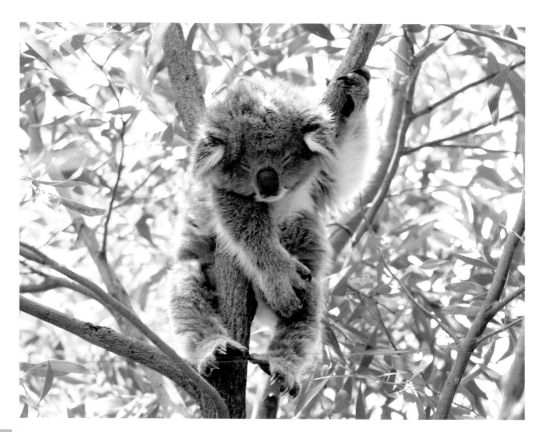

What Makes Eucalyptus Oil Special?

Eucalyptus oil is made up of a mixture of volatile compounds (volatile meaning that these fluids easily evaporate and turn into gases). The substance that gives eucalyptus oil its distinctive smell and taste is cineole, also known as eucalyptol. This is a clear liquid with a fresh fragrance and a spicy, cooling taste. But it has other properties: it is also antibacterial, a nasal decongestant, a respiratory anti-inflammatory, a cough suppressant and an effective solvent.

The other components of eucalyptus oil, such as pinene and limonene, have other health and practical properties, including antibacterial, antifungal, cleansing, disinfectant and deodorant ones. This combination of natural components, when extracted from the leaves, has a wide range of uses, which make a bottle of this clear oil invaluable. Eucalyptus oil, used on its own or with water and/or washing-up liquid, soap flakes or vinegar, can be used to clean anything from your clothes to the kitchen sink. It can also ease itching insect bites and aching feet, and help unblock noses.

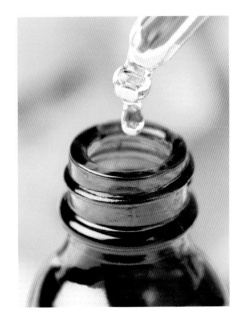

Health and Beauty

Eucalyptus has long been known for its health benefits – a powerful decongestant, it can bring wonderful relief to the miserable symptoms of a cold and other related illnesses. But its power extends far beyond that, showing signs of an ability to help with anything from bad breath to arthritis. It also has antibacterial and antifungal properties, which make it an ideal aid in the areas of health and personal care.

Around the Home

Eucalyptus has much more vastly unrealized potential – a powerful cleaning tool to be used around the home, eucalyptus gives both surfaces and laundry not only a thorough disinfecting but also an irresistibly fragrant and fresh smell. It can do a number of handy jobs around the home, from repelling insects to getting rid of dust mites and stopping dogs peeing on your car tyres.

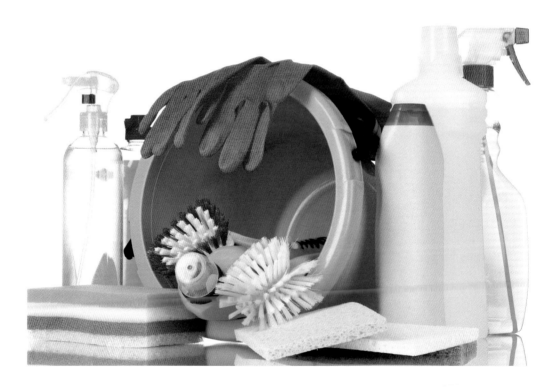

Doctor's Orders

While eucalyptus oil is very useful in many ways, there are some circumstances where you need to be careful – or even avoid it completely.

Eucalyptus oil is toxic if swallowed so make sure that the one you have at home is out of children's reach. Also, do not give cough drops that have eucalyptus in them to children under six. Do not put eucalyptus oil salve or rub on the face of any child under two years old. Be sure to check with your doctor before adding eucalyptus oil to hot water for a steam inhalation for children. The same applies to eucalyptus chest rub.

Don't swallow eucalyptus oil, even diluted, without your doctor's approval. It is toxic for adults as well as children. Like many other natural substances, it can interact with herbs, medicines and vitamins. Be particularly careful to talk to your doctor if you are on medication, as eucalyptus can change the way some medicines behave. Women who are pregnant or breastfeeding should also not use eucalyptus.

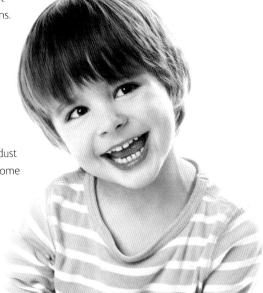

Although eucalyptus can be helpful for asthmatics (see the section on getting rid of dust mites), it can also trigger health problems in some people with this and other conditions. Don't use eucalyptus oil if you have asthma, liver or kidney disease, seizures or low blood pressure, without checking with your doctor first.

Be safe – and follow doctor's orders.

All About Eucalyptus

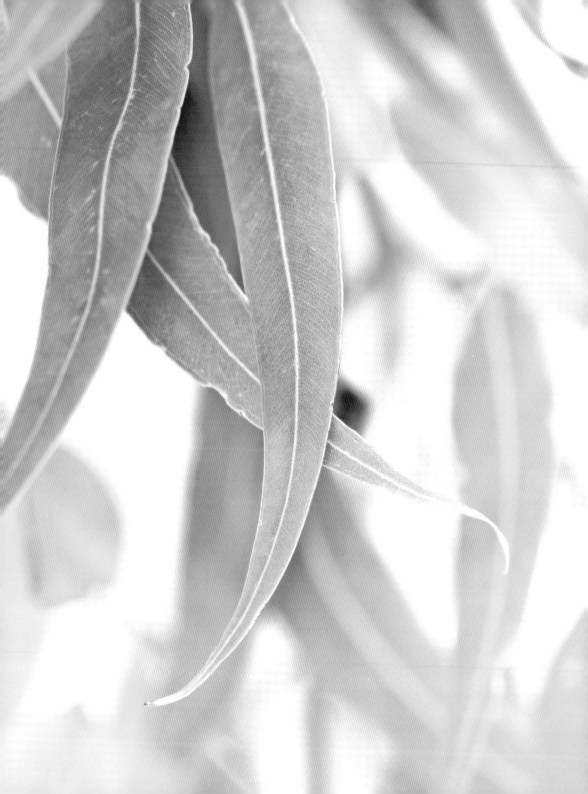

The Eucalyptus Plant

Eucalypts are extraordinarily useful and attractive trees, which are so adaptable that they can be found growing both in the freezing cold of the Snowy Mountains of New South Wales and in the heat of South America. As they are one of the fastest growing hardwood trees – in Brazil and Uruguay they can grow up to 6 m/roughly 20 ft in one year – they are an important source of timber for building, furniture and fuel. They are also, of course, the source of eucalyptus essential oil: a vital ingredient in any home.

Characteristics

What's in a Name

Eucalyptus plants come in different shapes and sizes, but the majority are very tall trees with large, leathery leaves. They are often called 'gumtrees', because of the thick, gum-like sap that oozes from the bark of some species. Other names are 'Scribbly Gum', due to the scribble marks left in the trunk of the trees by the larvae of tiny moths, and 'stringybark', because the bark can be pulled off the tree in long 'strings'.

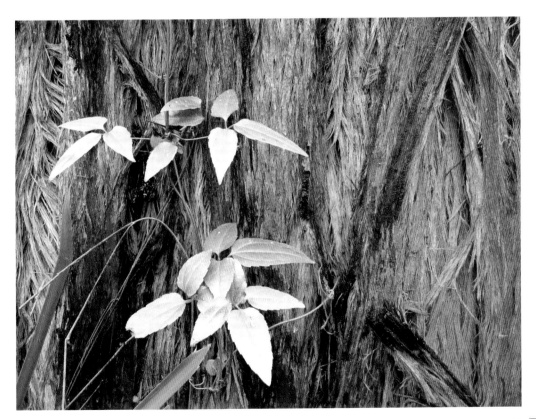

Colours

Many eucalypts shed their bark, displaying the different colours that lie beneath, on the bare trunk. There are many colourful species, with flowers of fuschia, coral, pink and white, and leaves of silver, grey and blue–green. Young leaves from the Tasmanian Blue Gum (*eucalyptus globulus*) are popular in floral arrangements.

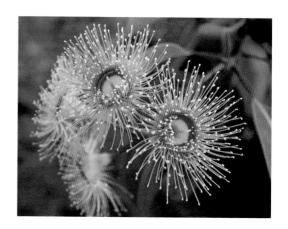

Fire

Due to the volatile oils in their leaves and flammable bark, these trees have evolved an unusual characteristic: they catch fire easily. Far from destroying them, the fire helps many varieties release their seeds. The ground beneath the tree, covered in ash from the fire, is ideal land in which the seeds can germinate.

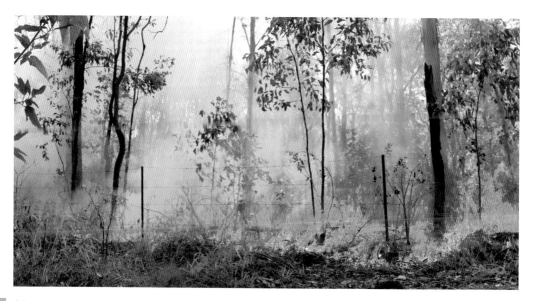

Water

The River Red Gum (or *eucalyptus camaldulensis*) also has the ability to suck up large amounts of water. It has been used to drain the water from swamps and rid the area of malaria-carrying mosquitoes. It is still used as a flood preventer and a soil stabiliser, as well as helping with reforestation.

Growing Tall

Eucalyptus trees range from the smallest – the Varnished Gum (*eucalyptus vernicosa*), which only grows to a maximum 4 m/13 ft high, and can be stunted to smaller than that – to the giant Mountain Ash (*eucalyptus regnans*), which can grow to 100 m/330 ft: almost as tall as Californian redwoods.

Eucalyptus globulus is one of the most popular varieties; it is planted in parks and gardens across Australia but also in many countries further afield, including India and Spain. It has white flowers and grey bark, which is shed in long ribbons.

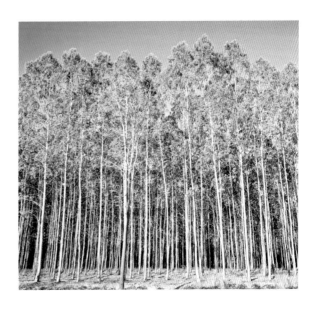

Eucalyptus pauciflora, also known as the Snow Gum, grows to a more manageable height of 8 m/25 ft, has white flowers and, when its bark sheds, its trunk is covered in attractive cream, grey and green patches.

Varieties

Vital Statistics

A good choice for a smaller garden in a temperate climate is eucalyptus preissiana, also known as the bell-fruited mallee. It has blue-grey coloured leaves, red-capped buds, stunning, large yellow flowers, and bell-shaped fruit. And, at a height of 2–3 m/ 6–10 ft, they are a more manageable size. There are many more varieties of eucalyptus, but before you set your heart on planting one in your garden, do check to see how tall they grow and what type of climate they need. As already mentioned, there are numerous different species of eucalyptus plants so here is a sample, complete with their vital statistics.

Corymbia Trachyphloia

Height: up to 25 m/82 ft
Spread: up to 10 m/33 ft
Also known as: Brown Bloodwood and *Eucalyptus Trachyphloia*

This species is fast-growing to a medium height and sheds its bark in short ribbons. It has white, sweetly scented flowers which, depending on the conditions, can be quite prolific.

Corymbia Maculata

Height: up to 30 m/98 ft
Spread: up to 20 m/65 ft

Also known as: Spotted Gum

It is closely related to two other species, *C. citriodora* and *C.henryi*, and they can be hard to tell apart when seen in their natural habitats. *Corymbia maculata* gets its spots from the patches of old bark that remain on the new, smooth powdery bark underneath, which is white, grey or pink.

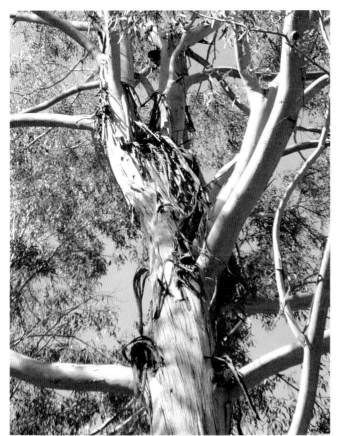

Eucalyptus Benthamii

Height: up to 25 m/82 ft
Spread: up to 20 m/65 ft
Also known as: Camden White Gum

The bark is shed from the upper trunk and branches of the tree in early summer, displaying the smooth white surface beneath. This is an endangered species in Australia and is named after an English botanist from the nineteenth century.

Eucalyptus Bridgesiana

Height: up to 20 m/65 ft (if not pruned)
Spread: up to 10 m/32 ft (if not pruned)
Also known as: Apple Box

It has a large, spreading crown and rough, fibrous bark on the trunk. The adult leaves are lance–shaped and dark or blue–green on both sides. It bears white flowers, usually in clusters of seven.

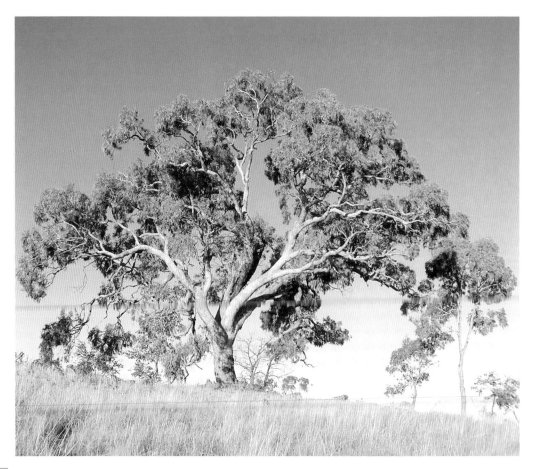

Eucalyptus Camaldulensis

Height: up to 8 m/26 ft (if not pruned)
Spread: up to 8 m/26 ft (if not pruned)
Also known as: River Red Gum

This is a fast-growing. hardy tree which can tolerate wet or dry soils and frost. It makes a useful windbreak and is good for providing shade.

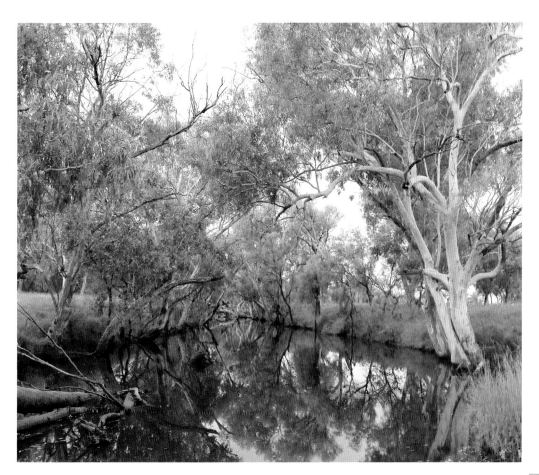

Eucalyptus Crenulata

Height: up to 6–12 m/20–40 ft
(if not pruned)
Spread: up to 4 m/13 ft (if not pruned)
Also known as: Buxton Gum, Victorian
Silver Gum

This is a fast-growing, relatively small tree
which tolerates shade. It responds well to
coppicing, so it's useful as a hedge or screen,
and it can also be grown in pots. It has a
smooth grey/yellow or grey/brown bark and
scented flowers.

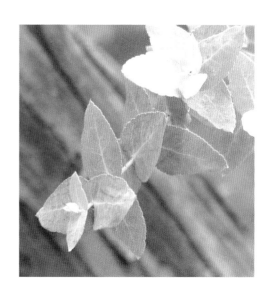

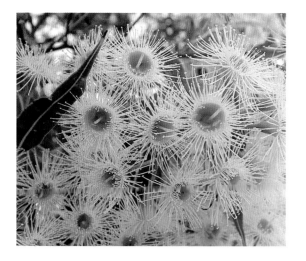

Corymbia Gummifera

Height: up to 30 m/98 ft
Spread: up to 8 m/26 ft
Also known as: Red Bloodwood

This fast-growing tree has glossy
dark leaves and clusters of attractive
cream/white flowers. It provides
good shade, fares well in most
soil types and doesn't need
much maintenance.

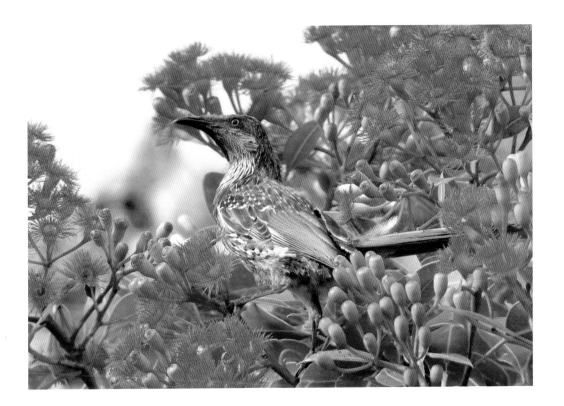

Eucalyptus Ficifolia (Corymbia)

Height: up to 7 m/22 ft (if not pruned)
Spread: up to 4 m/13 ft (if not pruned)
Also known as: Red-flowering Gum

This is a round, dense tree that makes a useful screen but is also attractive on its own.
It prefers soil with reasonable drainage and is moderately tolerant of frost. It has large,
bright red flowers.

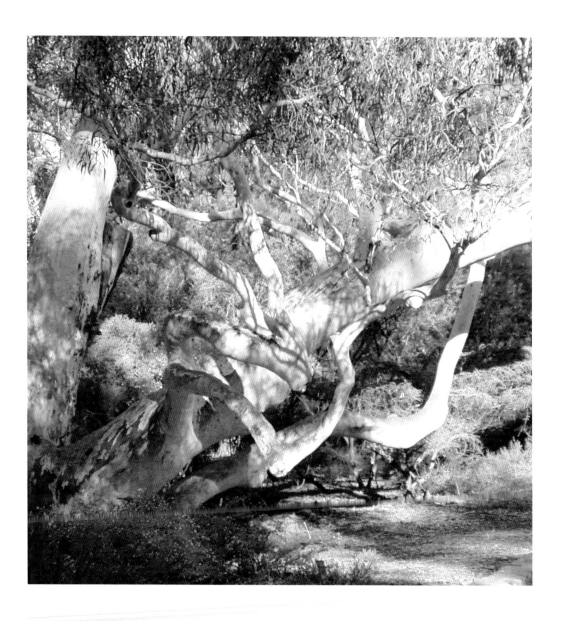

Eucalyptus Mannifera

Height: up to 20 m/65 ft
Spread: up to 5 m/16 ft
Also known as: Brittle Gum or Broad-leaved Manna Gum

Its smooth bark shreds in short ribbons or plates, showing the white, grey or red batches on the trunk of the tree. It has small white flowers and grey-green lance-shaped leaves. It is reasonably tolerant of drought and frost.

Eucalyptus Gunnii

Height: up to 10 m/32 ft (if not pruned)
Spread: up to 7 m/22 ft (if not pruned)
Also known as: Gum Tree, Ironbark

This is a fast-growing tree whose foliage is ideal for flower arrangements. The flaking bark reveals attractive patterns on the main trunk.

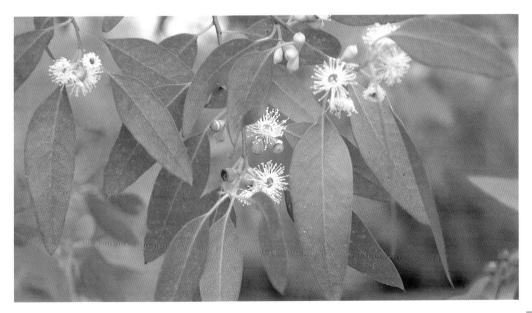

Eucalyptus Pulverulenta

Height: up to 10 m/32 ft (if not pruned)
Spread: up to 10 m/32 ft (if not pruned)
Also known as: Silver-leaved Mountain Gum

This is a slow-growing, easy-to-prune tree that can be shaped into an attractive bush, good for smaller gardens. It has silvery white/blue leaves, with a mass of creamy white fluffy flowers, and is popular with flower arrangers.

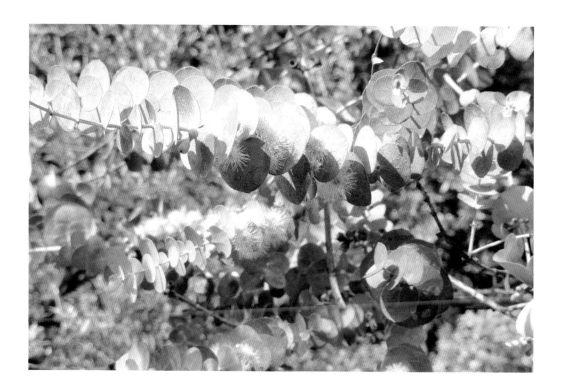

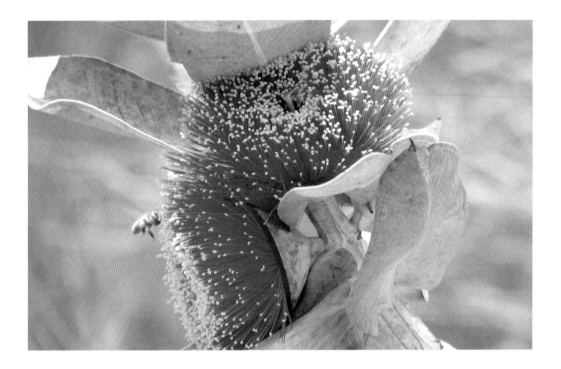

Eucalyptus Macrocarpa

Height: up to 4 m/13 ft (if not pruned)
Spread: up to 6 m/20 ft
Also known as: Mottlecah

These are very distinctive eucalypts, which grow like mallee varieties: with a number of shorter stems rather than one main trunk. They have spectacular red flowers, which can grow to be up to 100 mm (4 in) in diameter. They also have distinctive, and quite large, silver–grey leaves. These trees prefer climates that have a dry summer, and they can respond to quite hard pruning.

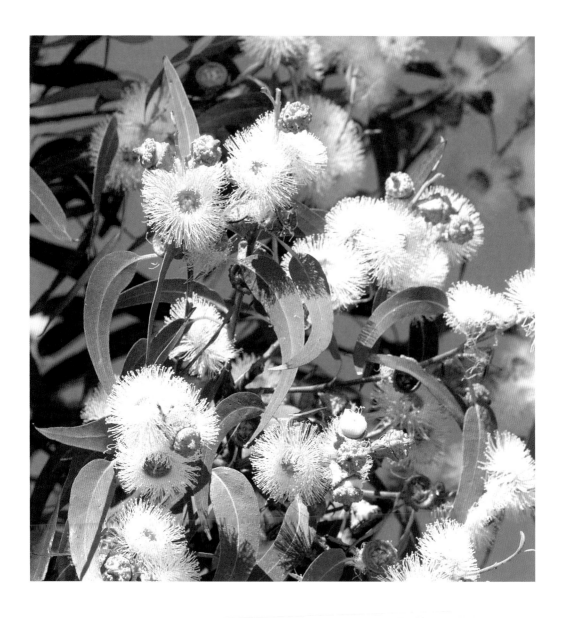

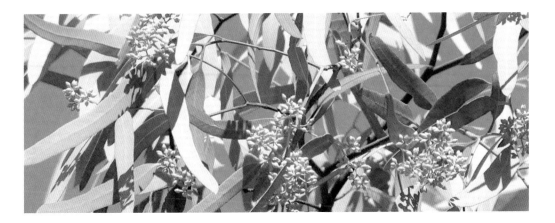

Eucalyptus Microtheca

Height: up to 10 m/32 ft
Spread: up to 7.5 m/25 ft
Also known as: Coolibah or Coolabah

This is a good shade provider which prefers well–drained, alkaline soil but is tolerant of heavy soil. Once established, it is also tolerant of drought.

Eucalyptus Globulus

Height: up to 20 m/65 ft (if not pruned)
Spread: up to 15 m/49 ft (if not pruned)
Also known as: Tasmanian Blue Gum

This spreading tree has a very fast growth rate and is tolerant of any type of soil; it is good at coping with frost and needs to be planted in full sun.

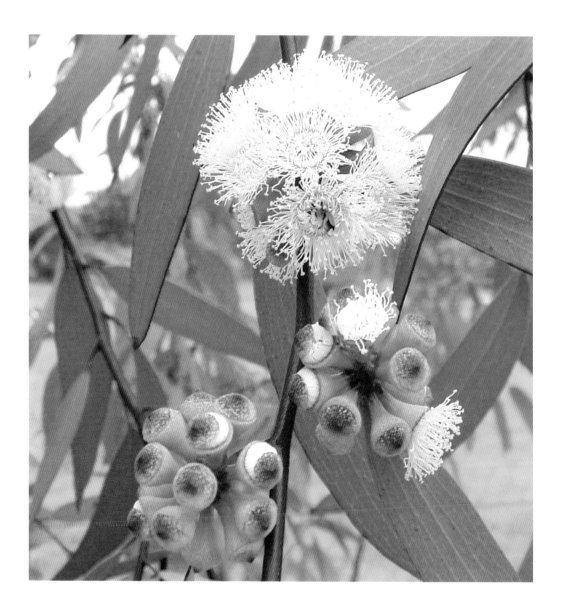

Eucalyptus Pauciflora Subspecies Niphophila

Height: up to 8 m/26 ft
Spread: up to 4 m/13 ft
Also known as: Snow Gum

It has green and grey/silver leaves; the young shoots are red and the flowers are white. The tree bark flakes to reveal a trunk with attractive grey, cream and green patches.

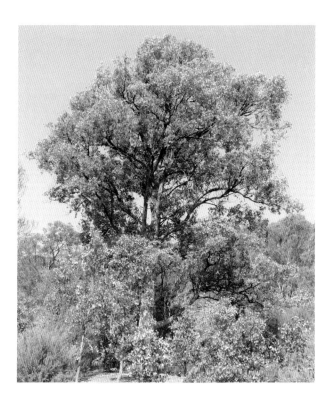

Eucalyptus Polyanthemos

Height: up to 20 m/65 ft
Spread: up to 15 m/49 ft
Also known as: Red Box

It grows well on dry, stoney soils with good drainage. This tree has leaves that are blue–green, coin–shaped and waxy with red veins. Relatively slow–growing, it responds well to pruning. It bears white flowers from early spring to summer.

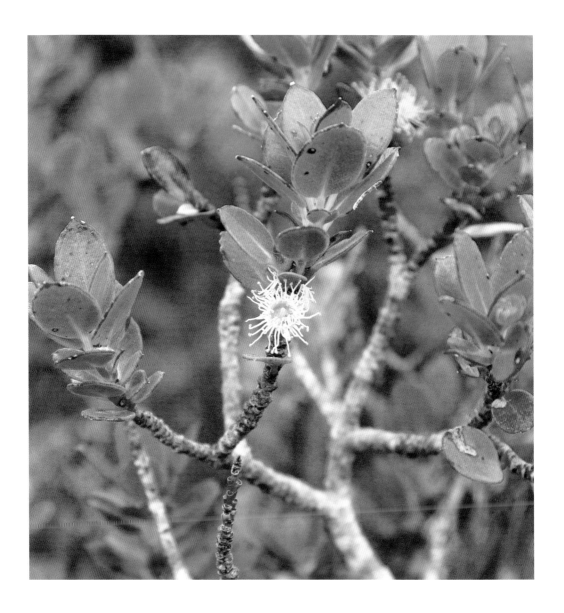

Eucalyptus Vernicosa

Height: up to 4 m/13 ft
Spread: up to 5 m/16 ft
Also known as: Varnished Gum

This plant has tiny glossy leaves, which give it its name of the Varnished Gum. It doesn't grow to be very tall, making it perfect for smaller gardens or even as a houseplant.

Eucalyptus Leucoxylon (Variant 'Rosea')

Height: up to 8 m/26 ft
(if not pruned)
Spread: up to 4 m/13 ft
(if not pruned)
Also known as:
Red Flowered Yellow Gum

This is a fast-growing medium-sized tree with masses of striking flowers consisting of numerous bright red/pink stamens, with long, sickle-shaped leaves. It suits soil with good drainage and full sun.

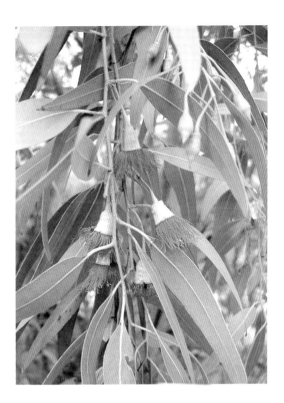

Eucalyptus Deglupta

Height: up to 75 m/246 ft
Spread: up to 24 m/79 ft
Also known as: Rainbow Eucalyptus, Rainbow Gum or Mindanao Gum

This species is famous for the colours it displays on its trunk. The rough bark sheds in patches, showing the inner, bright green bark which matures to stunning shades of blue, purple, orange and maroon. This tree is only suitable for outdoor growth in humid, cooler tropical temperatures and it does not tolerate freezing temperatures.

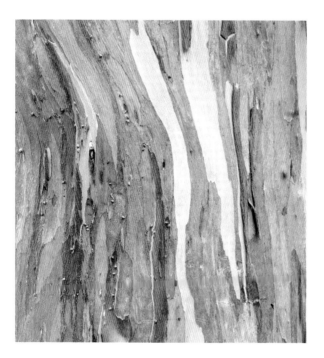

Eucalyptus Haemastoma

Height: up to 15 m/49 ft
Spread: up to 10 m/32 ft
Also known as: Scribbly Gum

The common name for this species (Scribbly Gum) comes from the wiggly lines left on its bark by the larvae of the scribbly gum moth. The diameter of the tunnel increases as the larvae grow in size. This species has smooth bark, glossy leaves and small white flowers.

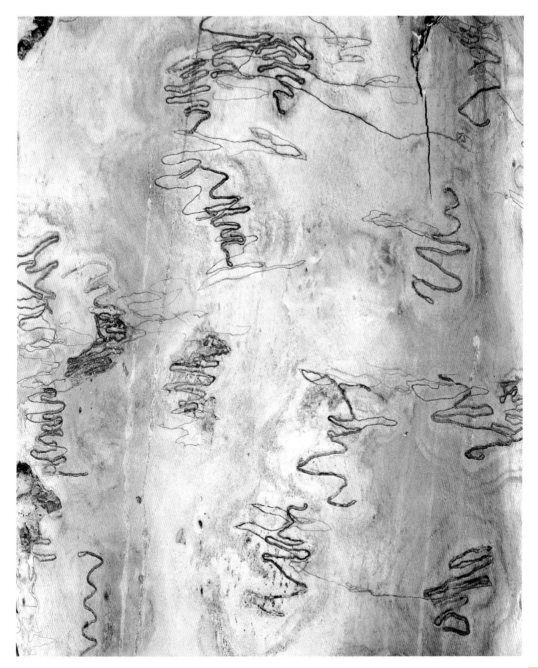

The History of Eucalyptus Oil

Eucalyptus has a relatively short history as far as its worldwide presence is concerned. However, when archaeologists started to dig deep, this remarkable plant shared some of its oldest secrets. In 2011, archaeologists working in Patagonia, South America, found eucalyptus fossils dating to 51.9 million years ago. These are the oldest authentic eucalyptus fossils found so far – and the only ones found growing naturally outside Australasia.

Origins

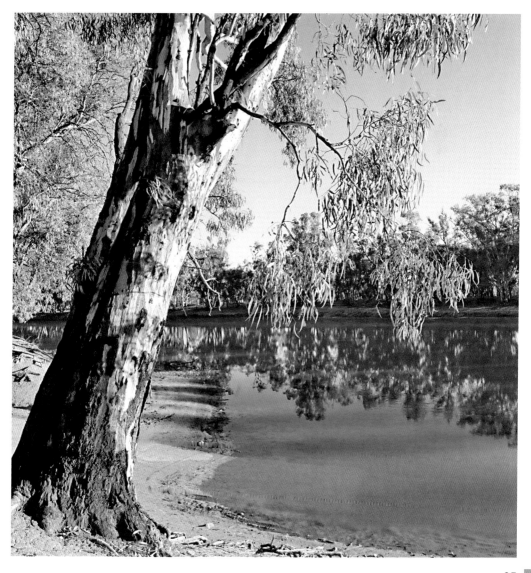

Aboriginal Beginnings

Skip forwards millions of years to find that eucalyptus has long been a part of daily life among the aborigines of Australia, Tasmania and a few nearby islands, where it is a native tree. The former were probably the first to realize that the oil from eucalyptus trees had health benefits and used it for healing and as an antiseptic.

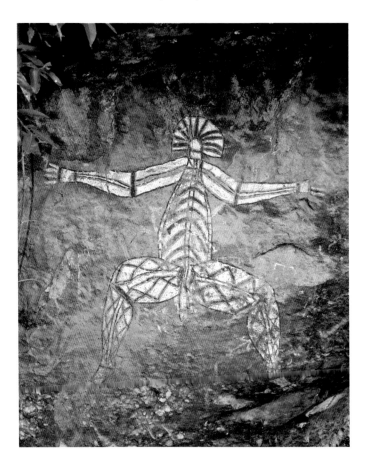

They used a number of different species to treat various ailments, including coughs, cuts, fever, diarrhoea and painful joints. They also traditionally used eucalyptus leaves to make infusions to treat pain, congestion and colds. Such knowledge was passed on through the generations. To the early British travellers to Australia, though, the benefits of eucalyptus oil were a completely new discovery – one which continues to be put to daily use around the world.

Western Discovery

News of this versatile tree and its wealth of properties useful to mankind only reached the Western world and beyond in the eighteenth century. It started with the arrival of the First Fleet in 1788, bearing amongst its passengers Royal Marines and their families, including children, along with civil officers and around 700 convicts.

With them came Surgeon–General John White, who, in his exploration of the land, noted that eucalyptus (then called Sydney Peppermint because of its minty scent) contained olfactory oil. He managed to extract some oil from the leaves and sent it to England for further study, where it was found to be more effective – and aromatic – than English peppermint, especially when dealing with 'colicky complaints'.

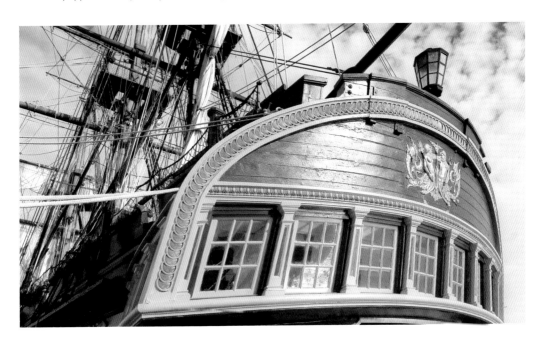

Joseph Bosisto

It wasn't until the arrival in Australia of another Englishman – Victorian pharmacist Joseph Bosisto, from Yorkshire – that the modern story of eucalyptus oil really took off. Bosisto started investigating the chemical and medicinal qualities of eucalyptus. He then built distilleries to extract the oil – and that is where it all started. He began supplying his essential oil to a small local market in 1852 and within a few years he was exporting it back to England.

By 1891 Bosisto had travelled around the world, displaying his essential oil at exhibitions, and by 1900 the eucalyptus oil industry had taken off: doctors were using this product to sterilize their equipment and to treat bronchitis, laryngitis, ulcers and other ailments.

Although Australia is no longer the dominant world supplier of eucalyptus oil (the rest comes from China, South Africa and South America), the original Australian Bosisto's 'Parrot Brand' eucalyptus oil is a popular brand today.

Production

Different Trees for Different Oils

Eucalyptus essential oil comes from the leaves of the plant and is extracted using steam. There are many different varieties of eucalyptus and, not surprisingly, they produce different types of oil. Only a few are suitable for commercial oil production, however, and fewer still produce oil that is suitable to be used in medicinal products.

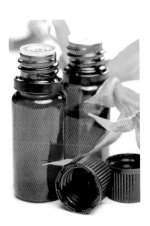

Crucial Cineole

One important factor to consider when choosing a variety of eucalyptus for essential oil production is picking one that has a high cineole content. Cineole is the colourless, oily liquid that gives eucalyptus oil its distinctive smell and taste. The essential oils from eucalyptus globulus, also known as 'the fever tree' because of its antiseptic qualities, and eucalyptus polybractea, both being varieties of eucalyptus with high cineole contents, are widely used for commercial purposes, particularly medicinal.

The Extraction Process

In order to extract essential oil from eucalyptus leaves, steam is forced through the leaf matter, thus vaporizing the oil. Once this is condensed, using cool water, the oil and water mixture separates, and the oil is collected and then refined. Australia was originally the leading producer of eucalyptus essential oil but has now been overtaken by China. Brazil and South Africa also produce eucalyptus oil commercially.

Laundry

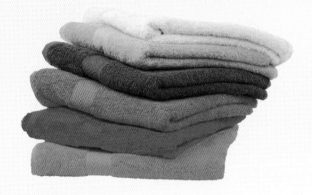

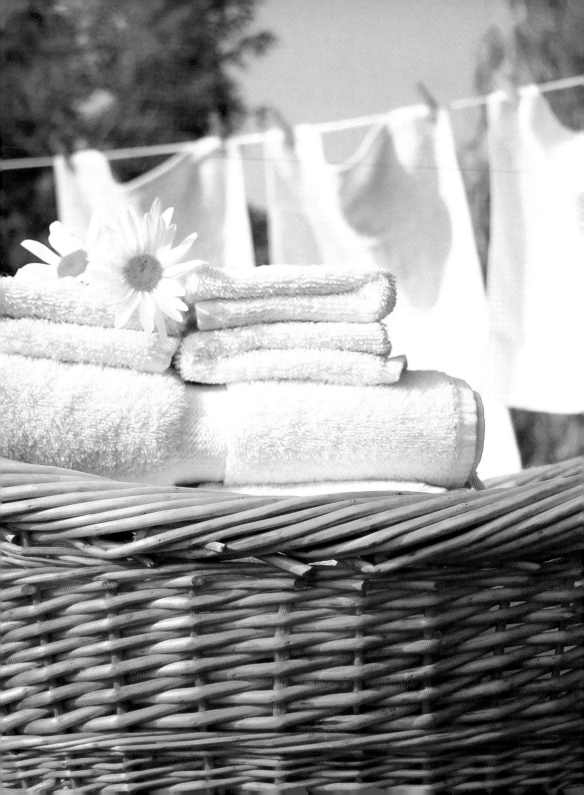

Cleaning

Eucalyptus oil has natural cleaning properties and, when used for washing, provides an effective addition to commercial washing liquids and powders. Eucalyptus essential oils do vary in quality, though, so it's important to check which country your oil has come from. The highest-quality oils are the most effective, and these are most likely to come from Australia and South Africa. As well as being a natural cleaner and disinfectant, eucalyptus oil is ecofriendly and thus doesn't introduce toxins into the environment.

Washing Clothes

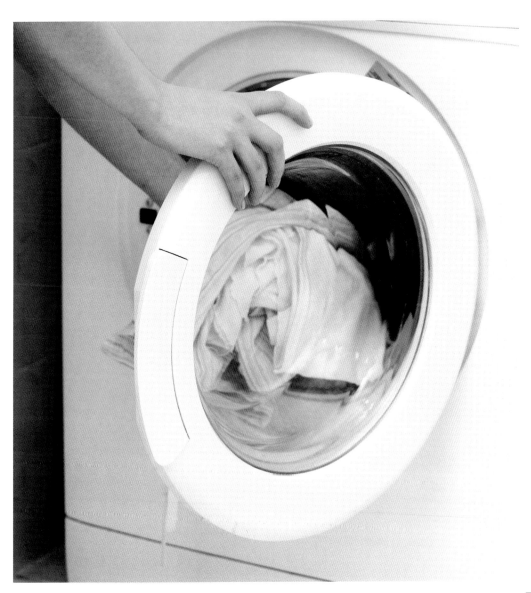

A Fresh Start

What better way to start the day than putting on clothes that feel clean and smell fresh! Inject some natural cleaning power in your wash by adding eucalyptus essential oil to your laundry; all you need to do is add 20 ml/¾ fl oz/1½ tablespoons to your machine wash.

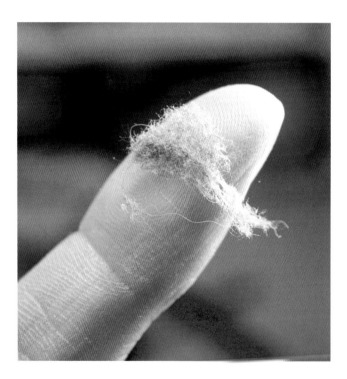

Dust Mites

These tiny creatures can be a problem for asthmatics, who therefore find it is essential to eliminate them from their clothes. Getting rid of them can often prove to be a real nightmare – but this could no longer be the case. Make a solution that is one part eucalyptus oil to 120 parts water and soak the clothes in it for about 30 minutes before washing them. They may smell of eucalyptus for a few days, but this will fade.

CAUTION: Research has found that eucalyptus oil can trigger asthma attacks in some people. Be particularly careful if there are young children in the house and if in any doubt, do not use.

Shirt Arms and Collars

The collars (where it touches the neck) and underarms are often the hardest part of a shirt to clean effectively. Spray them using a spray bottle with a mixture of 1 teaspoon eucalyptus oil for every 500 ml/18 fl oz/2 cups water. Concentrate on the most marked areas and if the fabric is very stained soak overnight using 1½ tablespoons in 4 litres/7 pints/16 cups warm water.

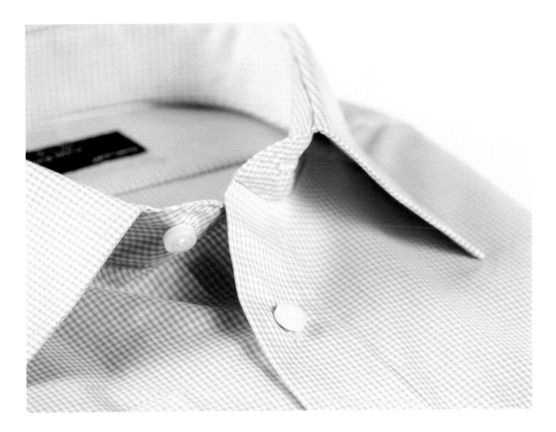

Deodorizing

If your clothes need a really good freshening up or are harbouring smells that won't go away, add a teaspoon or two of eucalyptus oil to your washing liquid when you do your laundry. You can adjust the amount *slightly* until you find the right mix for you. This natural deodorizer should help to remove those unpleasant odours.

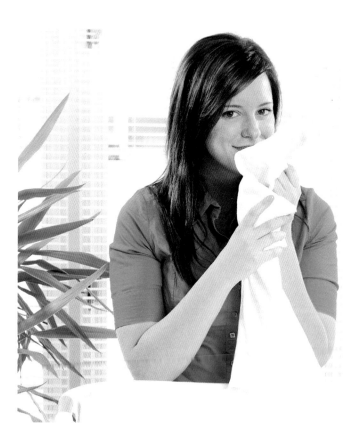

Disinfecting

There will be times when you need something really effective to deal with clothes or bedding that are particularly dirty or have been in contact with unpleasant substances. Thanks to its natural disinfectant properties, eucalyptus oil can help to solve the problem; simply add two capfuls of the oil to the water and soak the affected clothes for 30–40 minutes before washing.

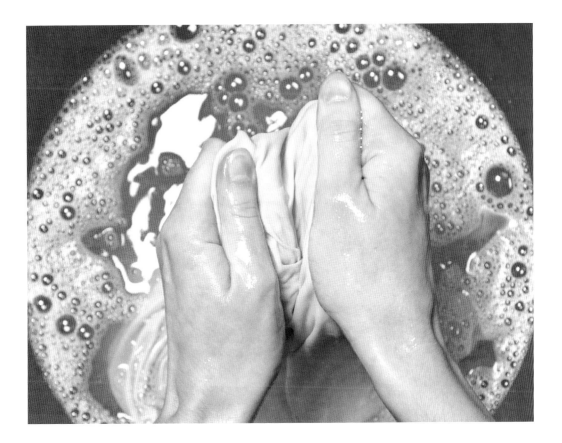

Handle With Care

When you have delicate items to wash, you may not want to entrust them to the washing machine. Add a small amount of eucalyptus oil – try half a teaspoon to start with – to your favourite hand washing liquid, and use warm, but not too hot, water. And remember to wash gently, as too much rubbing may harm the delicate fabric. Your clothes will be gently disinfected and will smell fresh and lovely.

Stain Removal

Pre-wash Spot and Stain Removal

A quick and easy way of boosting the cleaning and stain removing power of your wash is to make your own spray. Use a spray bottle – like the ones you use to spray water on to dry clothes before ironing – and add 1 teaspoon eucalyptus oil for every 500 ml/18 fl oz/2 cups water. Once this is done, simply spray the stained area of clothing before washing.

CAUTION: When using eucalyptus oil on clothing, always test to make sure that the fabric is colourfast. Do this by testing the oil on a piece of fabric that can't be seen when the clothes are worn.

Ink-stain Removal

Always finding ink stains from ballpoint pens on work or school shirts and other clothes? You can tackle them with eucalyptus oil. Put a clean, absorbent cloth underneath the stain, so it can soak up the ink, and then wet another clean cloth with drops of eucalyptus oil. Wiping carefully, you should be able to remove the stain. Once you've finished, you can wash the clothes as usual.

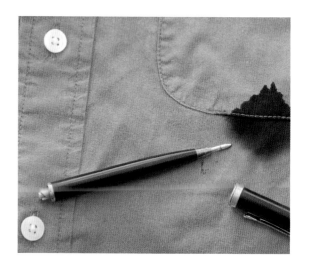

Grease Removal

When tackling grease spots and spills on clothing, just add 1½ tablespoons eucalyptus oil to your machine wash to get the best results. However, if any of the stain remains, use the same amount of eucalyptus oil in 4 litres/7 pints/16 cups warm water and leave the clothes to soak overnight before washing again.

Grass-stain Removal

Those bright green stains that come from playing or working out in the garden can take some removing, but there is an easier way to deal with them. Use a cloth damp with eucalyptus oil and, if possible, put a clean cloth on the underside of the stained fabric while you work on it. If you are tackling a persistent stain soak the clothing for an hour or more before you wash it.

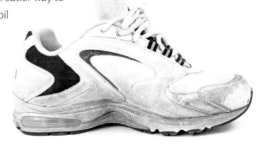

Tar Removal

This is a difficult substance to remove from clothing but, with a bit of patience, it should come off. Tackle the stain as soon as you can, as you'll find that wet tar is easier to remove than hard tar. Scrape as much of the substance off as you can by using the blunt side of a knife or similar item. Then put some drops of eucalyptus oil on a clean cloth or cotton wool ball, and wet the stain.

Place a clean, absorbent cloth underneath the stain and then, using a fresh cloth, remove what remains of the tar by working inwards towards the centre of the stain. As you do this, you may need to dampen the stain with eucalyptus oil again. Also, soaking the clothes in water mixed with washing liquid or powder may provide some additional help.

Conditioning

Eucalyptus is a really versatile addition to your laundry cupboard. It doesn't just make your washing smell fresh and invigorating, it also makes a difference to how your towels and woollen fabrics feel. Eucalyptus acts like a fabric conditioner and therefore it reinvigorates your fabrics, giving them a new lease of life and making them feel good to touch. And since it does all of this without putting harmful chemicals into the environment, you can feel confident that your washing is green as well as clean.

Fabric Softener

If you want to restore your clothes to their original softness why not try to make your own fabric conditioner rather than running to the shops to buy one? Add a few drops of eucalyptus oil to 250 ml/8 fl oz/1 cup white vinegar and place this mixture in the washing machine during the rinse cycle. You can add other oils, too, such as lavender, if you'd like to try a blend of scents.

Towels

Stepping out of the shower and wrapping yourself in a fresh, clean, soft towel is one of life's little pleasures. You don't need fabric softener to achieve this; just add two capfuls of eucalyptus oil to your wash and your towels will be fluffy and fragrant.

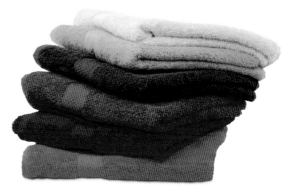

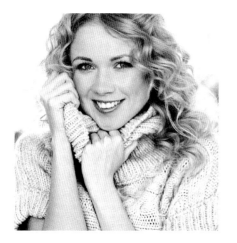

Woollens

Adding eucalyptus oil to your washing water is known to keep woollens soft, and it's easy to make your own washing liquid that's ideal for washing such garments. You need 500 ml/18 fl oz/2 cups soap flakes, 120 ml/4 fl oz/½ cup methylated spirits and 2 tablespoons eucalyptus oil. Pour them into a lidded jar and shake until they're thoroughly mixed together. When you next wash woollen items, add 2 tablespoons of the mixture for each litre/2 pints/4 cups warm water.

Cleaning

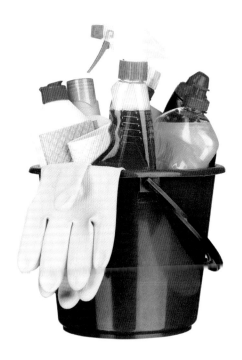

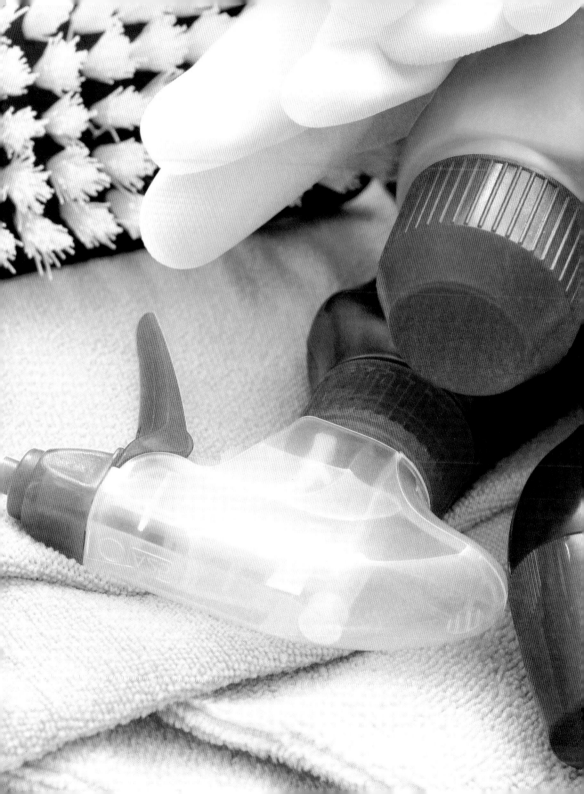

Kitchen & Bathroom

Eucalyptus oil makes a great addition to your cleaning tools. It is a natural disinfectant and antiseptic – laboratory studies have shown that eucalyptus oil contains substances that kill bacteria – and therefore ideal for use where good hygiene is important. The oil's clean, fresh smell also makes it a perfect deodorizer, which means it is the ideal choice for rooms like the kitchen and bathroom, which can need freshening up during the course of the day. Eucalyptus oil is also an effective cleaning agent and will work on a range of problem areas, including grease and mould.

Kitchen Items & Surfaces

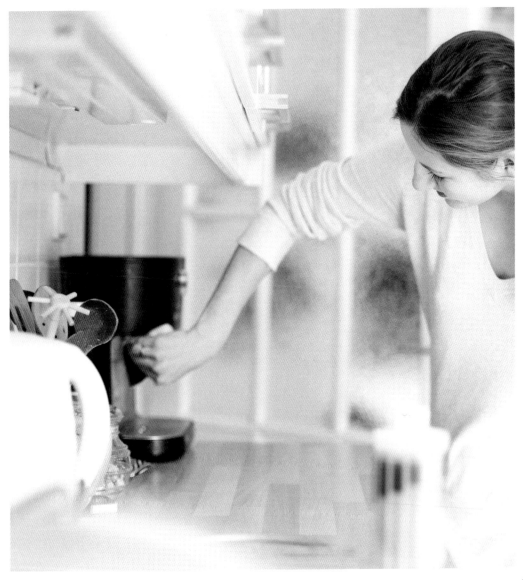

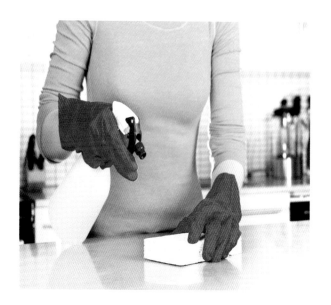

Gleaming Worktops

You can use eucalyptus oil to make an easy-to-use and effective cleaner for your worktops and other surfaces. Take a clean spray bottle and fill it almost to the top with water. Then add a small amount of washing-up liquid (a couple of short squeezes should do) and 2 teaspoons eucalyptus oil. Spray your worktops and wipe over with a clean cloth.

Kitchen Sink

The same mix of water, washing-up liquid and eucalyptus oil used to spray the worktops can be applied to coat your sink so that that, too, can be clean and disinfected. Once you've given the sink a good coating, wipe the mixture away with a cloth.

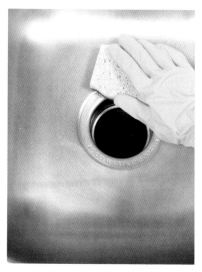

If your sink has a greasy residue and needs a really good clean, put the plug in and give it a good scrub with a sponge that has a scrubbing surface on the back. Then fill it with enough hot water to cover the greasy area and add washing-up liquid and five or six drops of eucalyptus oil. After leaving it to soak for a while, empty the water out and clean with a sponge.

Microwave

A mixture of two to three drops eucalyptus oil and 250 ml/8 fl oz/1 cup hot water can work miracles on your microwave, freshening it up and giving it a good clean. It can be applied to clean both the inside and outside of your microwave, but make sure you go over the inside with plain water afterwards. In order to remove stubborn food remnants from the inside, put a bowl of water in your microwave and heat for two minutes. Leave the door shut for another few minutes to allow the steam to loosen the stuck-on food.

Removing Grease

Making up your own grease-busting mix at home is easy and quick to do. First of all, pour water into a spray bottle until it's nearly full, and then add 2 teaspoons eucalyptus oil and a couple of squirts of washing-up liquid or liquid detergent. If you're tackling a particularly greasy area, such as the cooker hood or ceiling fans, try a mix with more eucalyptus oil; alternatively, pour eucalyptus oil on to a cloth and wipe the area that needs cleaning.

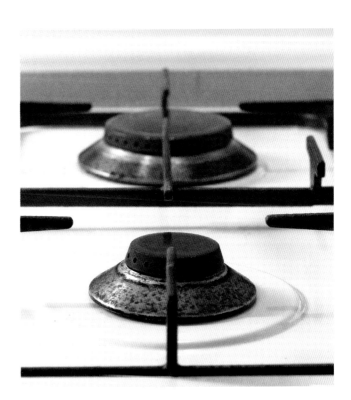

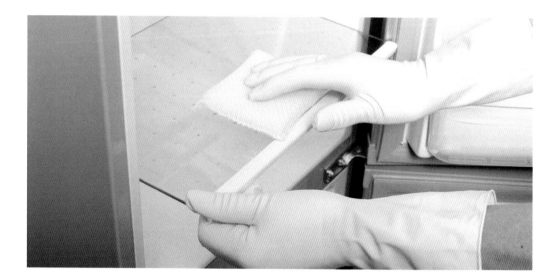

Fridge

Since eucalyptus oil has disinfecting and antiseptic properties, it's a helpful tool in the fight against mould. You don't need very much: just 250 ml/8 fl oz/1 cup hot water with a few drops of eucalyptus oil in it should be sufficient. Dampen a clean cloth with the water mixture and wipe down the inside of your fridge – and any other parts where you have a mould problem.

Dishwasher

These kitchen workhorses can often be forgotten in the hectic daily rush. However, with the help of some eucalyptus oil, it doesn't take long to clean and freshen them. Add a few drops of eucalyptus oil to some hot water and use this mixture to give the inside and outside of your dishwasher a thorough wipe. If there's any dishwasher soap that won't come off, wipe it off with some eucalyptus oil on a damp cloth. Wipe it all again with fresh water afterwards.

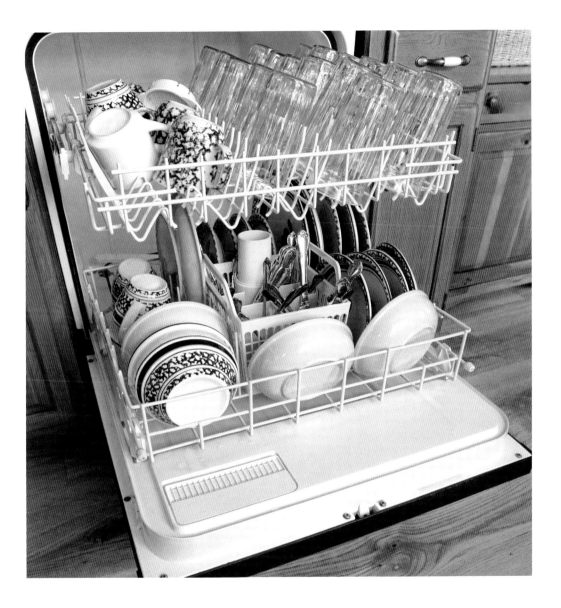

Odour & Pest Control

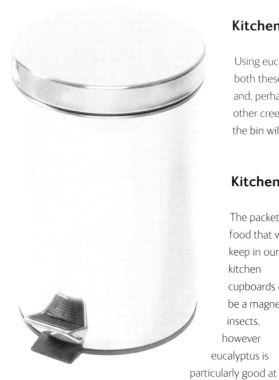

Kitchen Bin

Using eucalyptus oil in your kitchen bin will deal with both these jobs at once. Wipe the outside of your bin – and, perhaps, the area around it – to keep ants and other creepy-crawlies away. Also, a few drops of oil in the bin will leave it smelling fresh and fragrant.

Kitchen Cupboards

The packets of food that we keep in our kitchen cupboards can be a magnet for insects, however eucalyptus is particularly good at repelling them. Regularly give your cupboards a good wipe using a mixture of a few drops of eucalyptus oil and water. This should keep those uninvited guests away and it will also give your cupboards a clean, fresh scent.

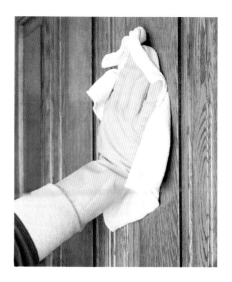

Bathroom

Floor Cleaner

The bathroom is one of those areas where you really want the floor to be clean. If your bathroom floor is a hard surface you can clean it effectively using warm water with a small amount of eucalyptus oil in it (2 teaspoons eucalyptus oil to half a bucketful of warm water). This mixture will give you a clean and disinfected floor.

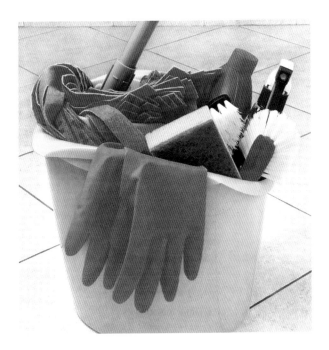

Tile Cleaner

Floor and wall tiles in the bathroom and shower can start to look quite grimy if not cleaned really regularly, but you shouldn't let this put you off. A mixture of 300 g/10½ oz soap flakes with 200 ml/7 fl oz/¾ cup methylated spirits and 50 ml/2 fl oz/¼ cup eucalyptus oil will give you the extra power you need to tackle the job. Rub the mixture on to the tiles and wipe clean; in some cases you may need to use a scrubbing brush. Then rinse with warm water and dry.

Shower and Bath Cleaner

You can use the simple warm water and eucalyptus mixture (2 teaspoons eucalyptus oil to half a bucketful of warm water) to clean your bath and shower regularly. If you prefer you can also add a few squirts of washing–up liquid. Wipe this mixture on to your bath and shower surfaces and then rinse off with clear water.

Scum Removal

We don't always have the time to clean the bath and shower every time we use them, and that can result in a build–up of soap scum on the surfaces. If that happens you might need

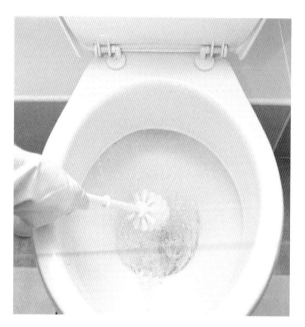

something stronger. Try mixing 300g/10½ oz soap flakes with 200 ml/7 fl oz/¾ cup methylated spirits and 50 ml/2 fl oz/¼ cup eucalyptus oil. Give surfaces a good clean and wash with plain water.

Toilet Cleaner

Eucalyptus essential oil is a good all–round cleaner and has disinfectant, antibacterial and deodorizing properties. These properties make it an ideal cleaner for your toilet. Add 2 teaspoons oil to the water in the toilet and clean with a toilet brush as you usually do.

Bathroom Vanity Units

Shampoo, conditioner, face cream, soap and toothpaste – all of these and more are stored in bathroom vanity units. And unless you're very careful, sticky marks can be left behind, which can trap dust and fluff, making the problem worse. Wipe the units clean with a cloth dipped in 250 ml/8 fl oz/1 cup hot water, with a few drops of eucalyptus oil in it. If there are any stubborn marks that won't shift, rub them with a cloth and a few drops of neat eucalyptus oil.

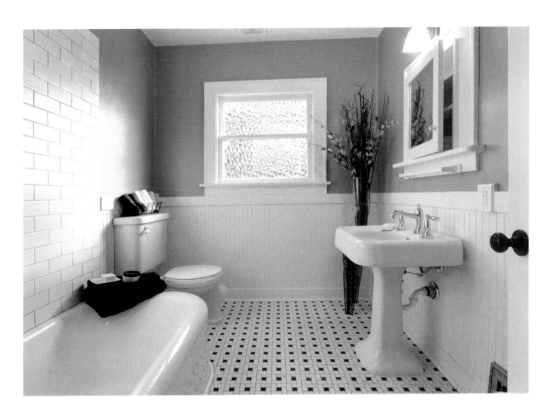

Bedroom

This is the place where you go for peace and quiet, for sleep and, when you're feeling unwell, for recuperation. Of all the rooms in the house, this is where you need to be able to find a sense of calm. Cleaning this room with eucalyptus oil will be a stress-free task, as eucalyptus is an efficient and green cleaner which won't bring unwanted chemicals into your haven. It will, however, leave your room smelling fresh and clean, and it will help to see off unwanted insect visitors

Linens

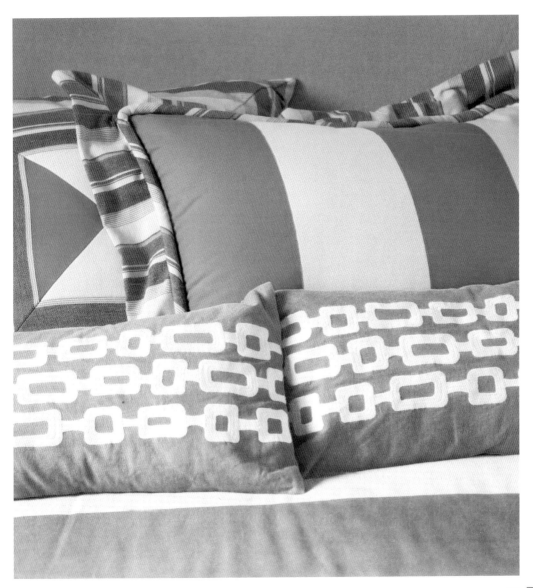

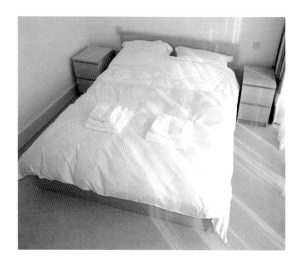

Fresh Sheets

Having fresh-smelling bed linens and bath towels can be the work of a few minutes. Spray a eucalyptus oil and water solution – 1 teaspoon eucalyptus oil for every 500 ml/18 fl oz/2 cups water – on to your bed linens before ironing or when almost dry (you can do this for towels and other such items too). Make sure all fabrics are dry before you put them away or use them.

Combat Dust Mites

Dust mites can get into our bed linen as well as our mattresses. However, there is no reason why you should have to put up with such unwanted pests, as there is an easy way to tackle them. Add eucalyptus oil to your wash – about 25 drops for each load – and then wash with liquid or soap flakes as normal.

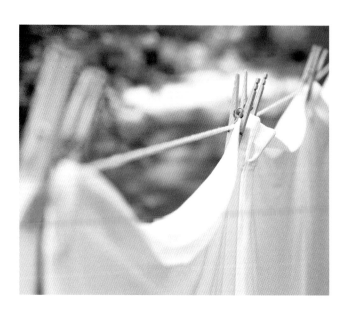

Furniture

Drawer Liners

When you open your bedroom drawers, you don't want to find moths and silverfish in there with your clothes. In order to keep your drawers smelling fresh and to ensure these pests keep out of them, wipe the liners and/or the drawers themselves with cloths which have been dunked in water and eucalyptus, and then squeezed to eliminate the excess liquid. A mix of 250 ml/8 fl oz/1 cup hot water and a few drops eucalyptus oil should do the job. Alternatively, you can use a few drops of eucalyptus oil on a clean cloth if you prefer.

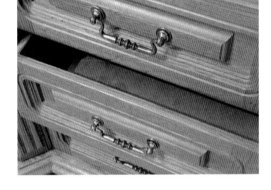

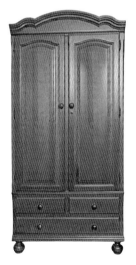

Wardrobes

In order to see off musty smells and moths, spray the inside of your wardrobe with a eucalyptus and water solution. Use a spray bottle – like the ones you use to spray water on to dry clothes before ironing – and add 1 teaspoon eucalyptus oil for every 500 ml/18 fl oz/2 cups water. You could also put a drop or two of eucalyptus oil on to a padded hanger.

Furnishings & Surfaces

Even in the most careful of homes, the inner fabric of the house – floors and counters, carpets and soft furnishings – can start to show the wear and tear of use over time. Eucalyptus oil, with its green cleaning properties, can be useful around the house in a wide variety of ways, without harming possessions or polluting the environment. Using natural products to keep homes and belongings looking their best has been a long-held tradition and is still a popular practice.

Stain Removal

Removing Chewing Gum

A piece of chewing gum stuck on any surface is enough to make your heart sink. However, you can remove this unpleasant chunk of rubbish from most surfaces with eucalyptus oil. Put a few drops of the oil on a clean cloth and rub on the chewing gum and surrounding area. You should have no trouble getting it off.

Ink, Grease and Grass

Carpets and upholstery can gather all sorts of nasty stains which can be very difficult to eliminate. Those caused by ink, grease and grass are particularly unsightly and can be stubborn to remove, however they can be removed very effectively by

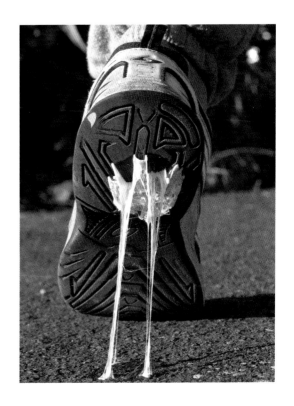

eucalyptus. Take a clean cloth and fold or scrunch it into a pad. Put enough eucalyptus oil on it to make the pad damp. Then, using the damp area, work the cloth on the stain, moving from the outside of it to the inside, so that you don't make the stain larger. Make sure that you carry out a patch test on a small, out-of-sight area first.

Floors

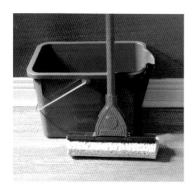

Wooden Floors

Make your wooden floors clean and hygienic by washing them with a water and eucalyptus solution. Just add a couple of teaspoons eucalyptus oil to half a bucket of water and mop your wooden floor as normal. An added bonus is that your floor will smell lovely too.

Lino

Eucalyptus oil works great on linoleum flooring too. Got some dirty marks on your lovely lino? Just mix up the same solution as described for cleaning wooden floors to clean and disinfect your linoleum floors. Mix 2 teaspoons eucalyptus oil to half a bucket of water and wash as normal.

Tiles

Tiles are a floor covering that can really show the dirt – especially if they're light coloured. However, using a mixture of 300 g/10½ oz soap flakes with 200 ml/7 fl oz/ ¾ cup methylated spirits and 50 ml/2 fl oz/¼ cup eucalyptus oil should deal with all your grubby floors. For a lighter wash, add 2 teaspoons eucalyptus oil to half a bucket of water and wash as usual.

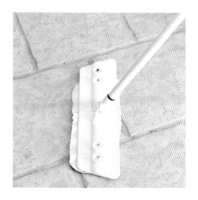

Scuff Marks

Eucalyptus essential oil can make short work of scuff marks on most floors. Mix together 1 teaspoon eucalyptus oil for every 500 ml/18 fl oz/2 cups water and put the resulting solution in a spray bottle. All you need to do now is squirt the scuff mark and rub with a cloth. However, if the scuff won't shift, tip a few drops of eucalyptus oil on to a cloth and wipe the mark off.

Vacuum Cleaner

A few drops of eucalyptus essential oil in your vacuum cleaner bag – or on the filter – can make a pleasant difference to your cleaning regime. The essential oil in the bag can help to kill off any creepy–crawlies that get sucked in there. And the oil on the filter can add a fresh fragrance to your home.

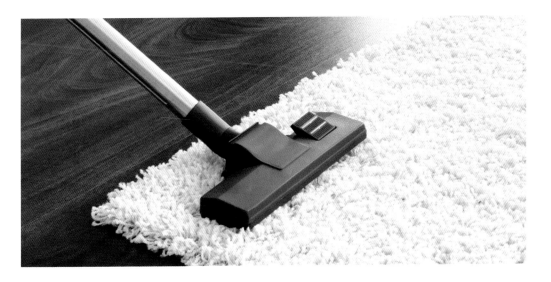

Surfaces

Windows

In order to get your windows sparkling clean, make up your own mix of window cleaning solution. Use 250 ml/ 8 fl oz/1 cup white vinegar and add five drops of eucalyptus oil. Put in a spray bottle, squirt it on your windows and then wipe them with a clean cloth.

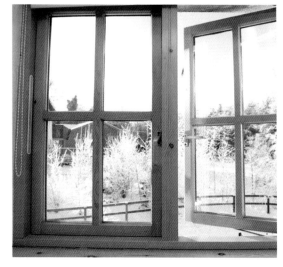

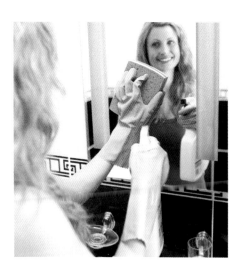

Mirrors

Give your mirrors a good spring clean with a home-made cleanser. Put 250 ml/8 fl oz/1 cup white vinegar and five drops of eucalyptus oil into a spray bottle. Squirt your mirrors with this mixture and wipe dry with a soft cloth. And there's an added benefit: this mixture reduces mirror fogging after baths and showers so you'll still be able to see yourself.

Leather

Leather items, such as shoes, bags and sofas, are usually quite an investment, so getting any marks out without causing further damage to them is likely to be a priority. This can be easily achieved by carefully wiping over the marked area using a clean, damp cloth with a few drops of eucalyptus oil added to it.

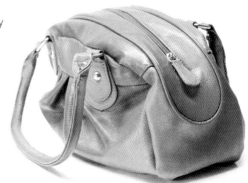

CAUTION: Make sure you do a patch test first on an area that can't be seen.

Plastic and Vinyl

Eucalyptus oil can clean ink and other stains off many types of plastic and vinyl – for instance, plastic book covers and stationery items where a pen has leaked. Use 1 teaspoon eucalyptus oil for every 500 ml/18 fl oz/2 cups water to start with. However, if the marks prove stubborn, try a few drops of undiluted eucalyptus oil on a cloth.

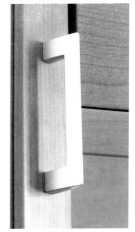

CAUTION: Always do a patch test on an area of the plastic or vinyl that can't be seen first.

Stainless Steel

You want the stainless steel items in your home – from your cupboard handles to your fridge – to look clean and smart. Mix a teaspoon eucalyptus oil in to 500 ml/18 fl oz/2 cups water and use this solution to wipe away those sticky finger marks.

General Household

As our lives become busier and more pressured, finding a quick, simple and yet effective way to deal with everyday tasks becomes ever more crucial. Keeping our homes and workplaces clean is important to our self-respect, but finding the time to do these jobs isn't always easy. Eucalyptus oil, with its cleaning and disinfecting properties, holds the answer to this dilemma. Its simplicity of use and ability to tackle many different jobs make this versatile liquid a household essential.

All-purpose Disinfectant

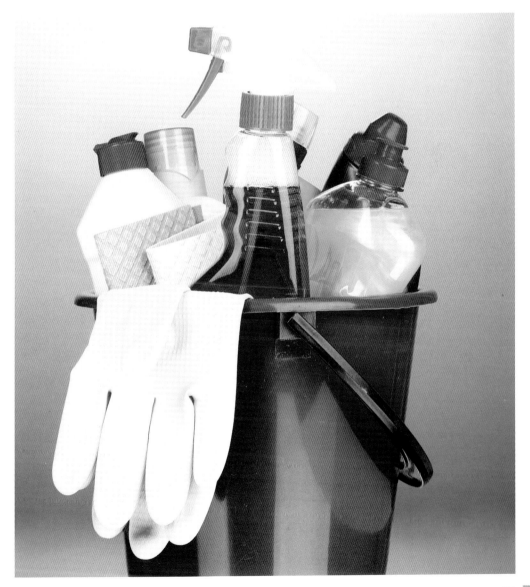

Phones

When the phone goes, we tend to grab it quickly and often end up smearing it with whatever we've just been touching, from butter to ink or worse. In order to clean and disinfect your phone, wipe it with a clean cloth that has a few drops of eucalyptus oil on it. Next time you use it, it will smell good, too.

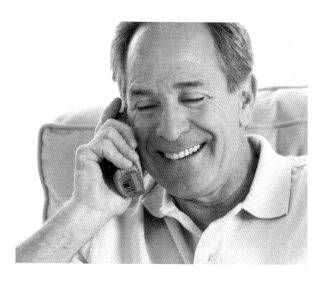

Keyboards

They're a vital part of your computer, but they're notorious for being a breeding ground for bacteria. In order to clean and disinfect your keyboard, first of all unplug it from your computer (or unplug your computer) and then dust it with a soft brush. Once this is done, wipe the keyboard gently with a cloth sprayed with a mixture of 1 teaspoon eucalyptus oil in 500 ml/18 fl oz/2 cups water.

Central Heaters/AC Unit Filters

When you wash your central heating and air conditioning filters, you should rinse with clean water after using soapy water. By adding 2 teaspoons eucalyptus oil to the clean water you will make the most of the oil's disinfecting and deodorizing properties.

CAUTION: Make sure you read the central heating and air conditioning manufacturers' instructions before you start.

Door Handles

Think of how many times door handles are used every day. The opportunities for making them grubby – and riddled with germs – are endless. However, there is a simple way to clean and disinfect them in one go. Wipe with a cloth dampened with eucalyptus oil and make those handles nicer to touch.

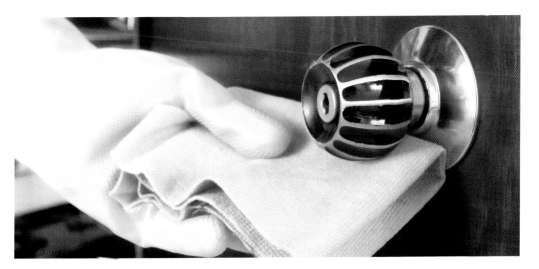

Residue Remover

Stickers and Price Labels

These adhesive-backed stickers and labels can leave behind a residue that looks messy and gathers dust, hairs and other dirt. Get rid of these marks easily with a spray of eucalyptus oil and water (1 teaspoon eucalyptus oil for every 500 ml/18 fl oz/2 cups water) or wipe with a cloth and a few drops of eucalyptus oil, and leave for a little while before wiping away.

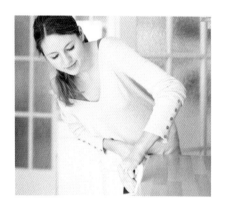

Sticky Finger Marks

You can often tell where small children – and big ones – have been in your home by the trail of sticky finger marks they leave behind. Clear these away by spraying them with a mixture of 1 teaspoon eucalyptus oil in 500 ml/18 fl oz/2 cups water. Simply put this solution into a spray bottle, squirt and wipe off.

Bandages and Plasters

Sticking plasters and bandages are a great way of covering cuts and helping to keep them clean, but the gluey bits left behind when the bandage or plaster comes off can be a nuisance to remove. Dampen the sticky residue with eucalyptus oil on a cotton wool ball or cloth and it should come away easily.

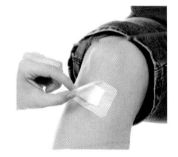

Odour

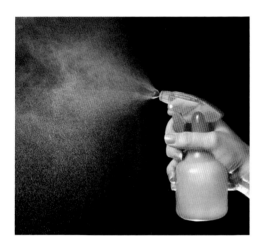

Air Freshener

All homes and workplaces develop a stale, musty smell from time to time. In order to change this to a fresh, invigorating scent, spray the rooms and hallways with eucalyptus oil and water. Prepare a mixture of 1 teaspoon eucalyptus oil for every 500 ml/18 fl oz/2 cups water and put into a clean spray bottle to use.

CAUTION: Eucalyptus oil is flammable so do not use near flames.

Bins

Rubbish bins, large and small, can quickly start smelling unpleasant if they aren't cleaned on a regular basis. Make this job easier by spraying them with eucalyptus oil and water (1 teaspoon eucalyptus oil for every 500 ml/18 fl oz/2 cups water, in a spray bottle). Alternatively, add 2 teaspoons eucalyptus oil to half a bucket of water, pour into the bin and wipe with a cloth or mop.

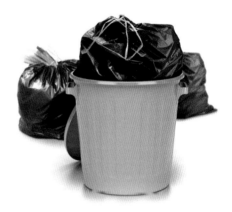

Animals

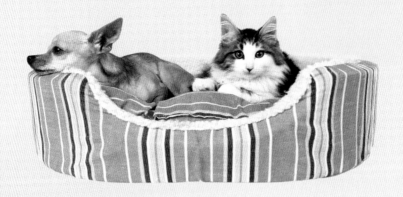

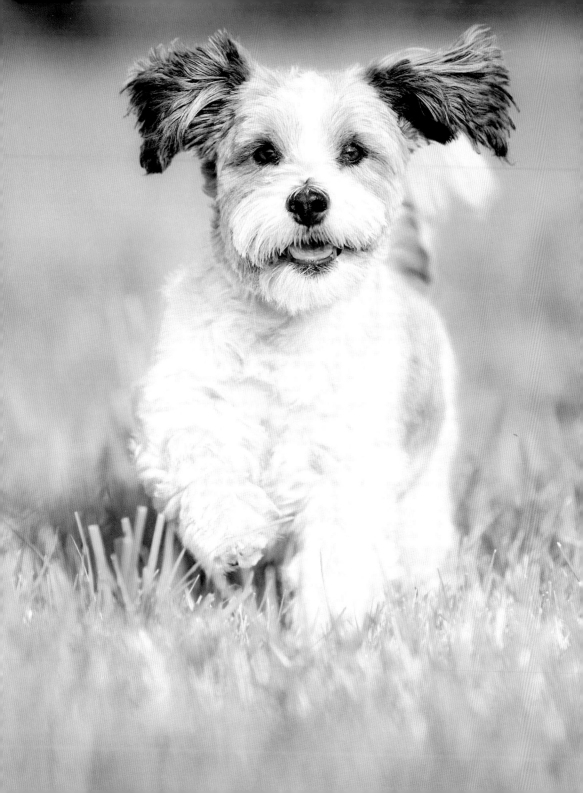

Pet Care

With a bottle of eucalyptus oil in your cupboard you'll be equipped to tackle many aspects of caring for your pets, from keeping their bedding clean and fragrant to ridding them – and your home – of fleas. A small amount of eucalyptus oil added to water and other cleaning and washing items can achieve a great deal, including making your home fresh, disinfected and sweet-smelling. Here you will find some simple ways in which you can solve some of the common cleaning issues most pet owners have to face.

Cleaning Up

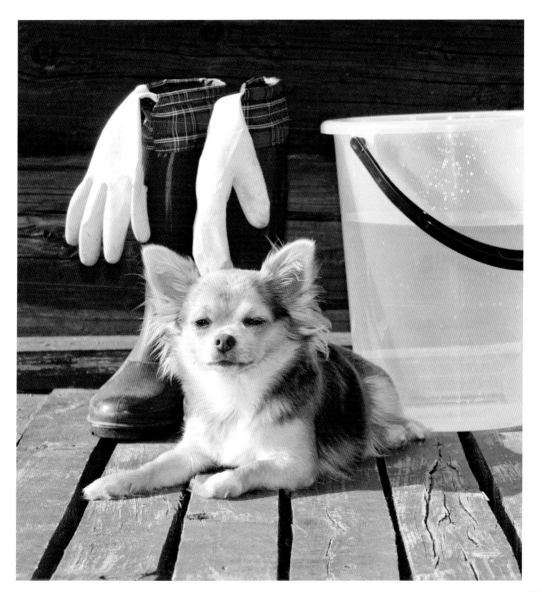

Be Careful

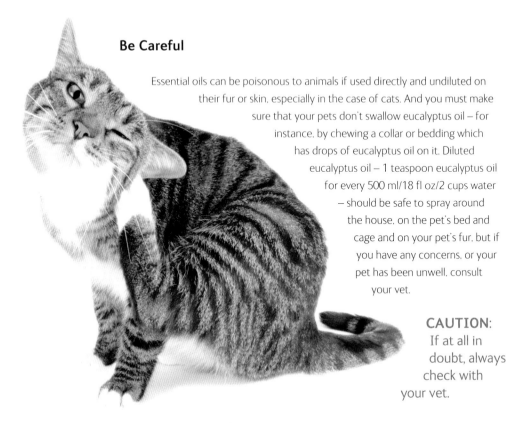

Essential oils can be poisonous to animals if used directly and undiluted on their fur or skin, especially in the case of cats. And you must make sure that your pets don't swallow eucalyptus oil – for instance, by chewing a collar or bedding which has drops of eucalyptus oil on it. Diluted eucalyptus oil – 1 teaspoon eucalyptus oil for every 500 ml/18 fl oz/2 cups water – should be safe to spray around the house, on the pet's bed and cage and on your pet's fur, but if you have any concerns, or your pet has been unwell, consult your vet.

CAUTION: If at all in doubt, always check with your vet.

Wipe Your Paws

Much as we love our pets, they can make our homes smell a little fusty – or worse. And, being animals, they don't bother wiping their feet when they come in, so any germs they walk in get trodden all over our rooms. Eucalyptus oil can help to disinfect and deodorize your home, all in one go. Add two caps of eucalyptus oil to your hot water when cleaning floors, doors and other surfaces. For particularly grimy areas, use a few drops of eucalyptus oil on a clean cloth.

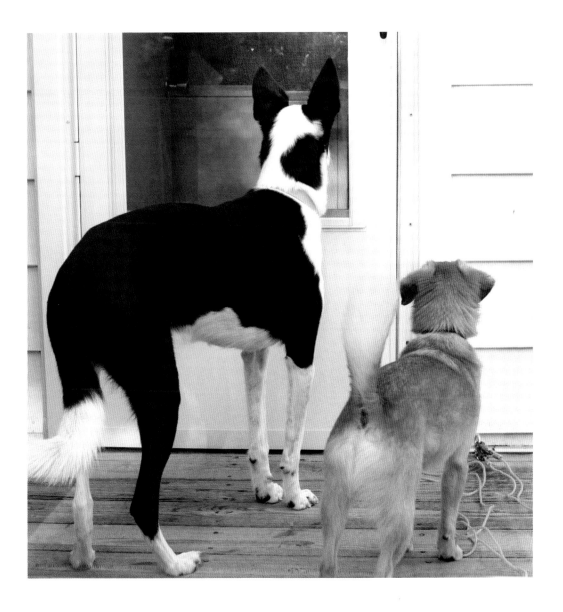

Dog Shampoo

A simple way of making a flea repellent for your dog is to add scant ½ teaspoon eucalyptus oil to about 2½ teaspoons of your normal dog shampoo. Wash the dog with the shampoo as usual, then wash all the shampoo off and dry your dog. If your dog has sensitive skin, ask your vet before using.

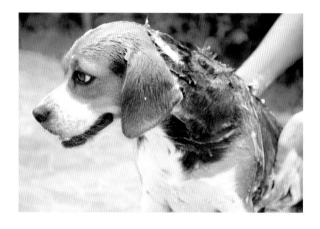

You may also want to try just a small amount of eucalyptus oil/shampoo first. Alternatively, you could make a eucalyptus spray using 1 teaspoon eucalyptus oil for every 500 ml/18 fl oz/2 cups water.

CAUTION: Do not use this shampoo on cats. Cats are especially sensitive to essential oils and eucalyptus oil must not come into direct contact with their fur or skin.

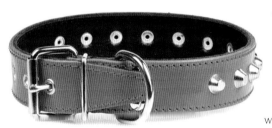

Goodbye Fleas

Another handy tip for keeping those pesky fleas at bay is to put a few drops of eucalyptus oil on your pet's collar. This is particularly useful for cats who can't be washed with the flea-repelling shampoo, but can apply to any pet with a collar.

CAUTION: Don't do this if your pet is prone to chewing their collar.

Little Accidents

Sometimes your pets have a little accident on the carpet. Instead of putting it off, try to deal with this when the urine is still wet. Mop it up thoroughly, using paper towels or something similar, soaking up as much of the liquid as you can. Then, using a spray bottle, spray the affected area with a mix of 1

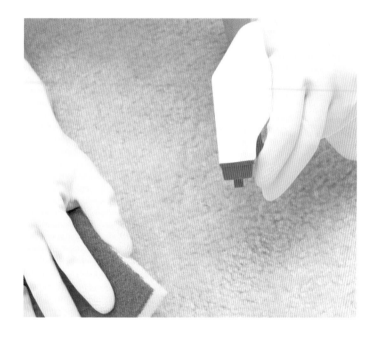

teaspoon eucalyptus oil for every 500 ml/18 fl oz/2 cups water. Mop thoroughly and repeat, mopping again. A variation on this mixture is to add some white vinegar and some washing-up liquid.

Masking the Smell

It's important to get rid of – or mask – the smell of urine because otherwise your pet will return repeatedly to the same spot to wee on it again. Using the eucalyptus oil and water spray mixture used for cleaning urine from the carpet should remove the smell too. You can try making the mix with more eucalyptus oil if this doesn't work straightaway, but always do a patch test first to check for colourfastness. Pets often aren't keen on the smell of eucalyptus, so this may also help to keep them away.

Health & Wellbeing

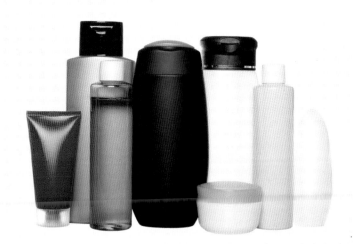

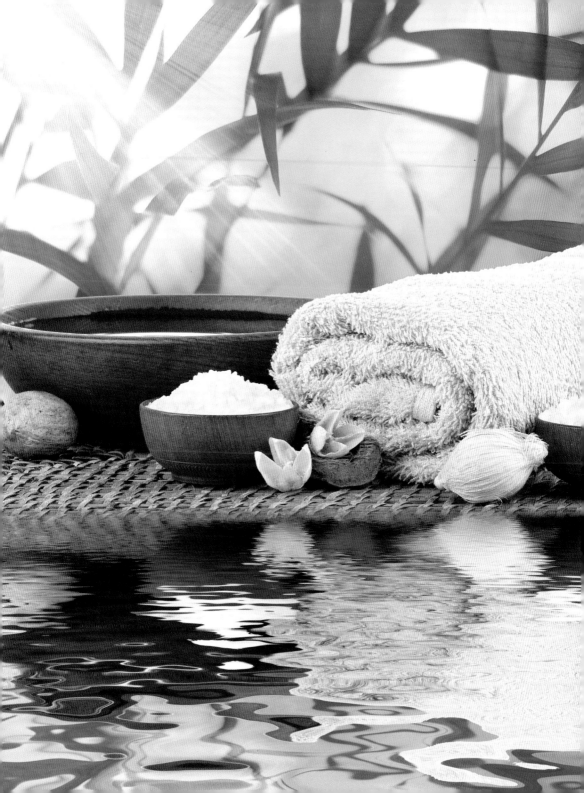

Appearance & Wellbeing

Since eucalyptus oil has so many properties related to wellbeing, it's not surprising that it has, for many years in the past, often been used in lotions, shampoos and soaps. Its continued popularity is clear from the availability of products containing eucalyptus in shops and online. You can, however, make your own eucalyptus oil preparations at home. By doing this you can be sure that the ingredients are environmentally friendly, and you will also get the chance to tailor the ingredients to your own tastes and requirements.

Skin

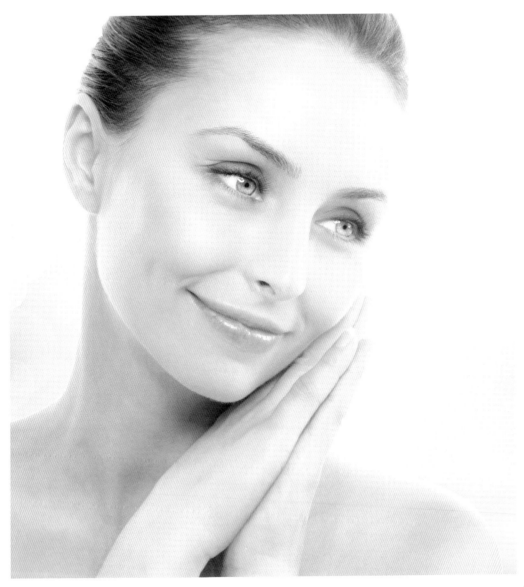

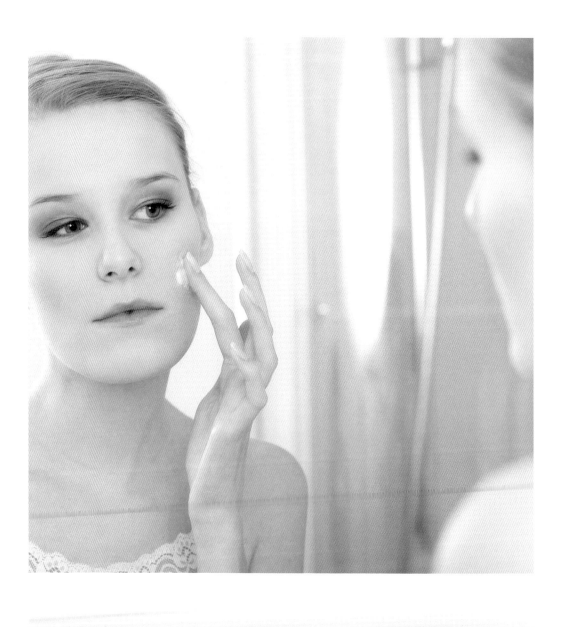

A Word of Warning

Talk to your doctor before you use eucalyptus oil if you have asthma, seizure disorders or liver or kidney disease, or if you are pregnant or breastfeeding. You should not give it to children aged two and under, and you should seek medical advice before using it on or near children aged 12 and under. Some of the sections in this book contain recipes and uses of eucalyptus oil that are believed to be beneficial for people suffering with asthma; however, some asthmatics can have adverse reactions to the oil. If you, or a family member, have asthma and eucalyptus oil is a trigger for an attack, do not use it without taking medical advice.

Face Lotion

A small amount of eucalyptus oil added to a base oil makes a lotion that can be used in a variety of ways. Since eucalyptus has natural antibiotic and anti-inflammatory properties, it may help adults with acne. However, you should always check with your doctor or dermatologist before using a home-made treatment containing essential oils. This is particularly important if you are already taking medications of any kind.

Measure out 120 ml/4 fl oz/½ cup base oil, such as almond or olive oil, and mix in 8 drops of eucalyptus oil (see CAUTION below.) Before you go to bed, use a cotton bud or some cotton wool to gently dab the lotion on to the areas of your skin affected by acne. Always take care when using eucalyptus and other essential oils. Essential oils are very concentrated and must be diluted before you use them, unless your doctor has advised otherwise.

CAUTION: Be careful not to get lotion containing eucalyptus oil – or neat eucalyptus oil – into your eyes, nose or mouth, and do not use it on children, especially those aged under two years.

Skin Patch Test

Before you use a eucalyptus oil face lotion – whether it's one you've made yourself or one you have bought – make sure you always do a skin patch test. If you're making your own by adding eucalyptus oil to an existing cream, take some of the base lotion – about the size of a grape – and add one drop of eucalyptus oil to it. Then rub a small amount on to your inner forearm – make sure it's clean and dry, and that it doesn't have any other lotion on it already. Then wash your hands.

Leave it for 24 hours and check to see whether you have had an adverse reaction. If it's alright, the eucalyptus lotion should be fine to use. But don't use too much of it and don't use it on large areas of skin. If you have had an adverse reaction you may notice this before the 24 hours are up. In this case, wash the area of the patch test and dry carefully. If you feel ill or have serious symptoms get medical advice as soon as you can.

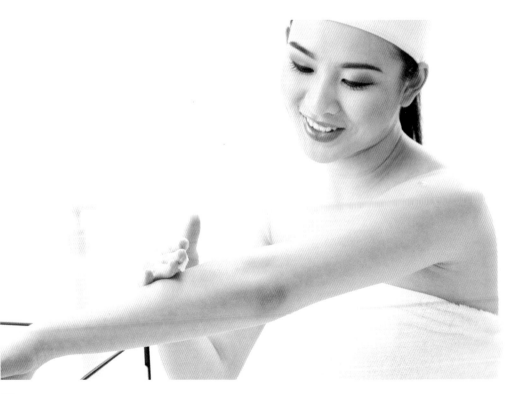

Clean Hands

If you want to make yourself a hand wash, add 1 teaspoon eucalyptus oil to 50 ml /2 fl oz /¼ cup warm water, stir well and pour on your hands to wash. You can make this mixture in larger amounts, but don't make more than you need.

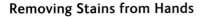

Removing Stains from Hands

If you've been spring–cleaning, working on the car or decorating and can't shift paint, oil or other stains, slightly moisten a clean cloth with a few drops of eucalyptus oil. Then wipe the stains away – they should go without too much effort – and wash your hands with soap and water as you normally would. If you have an adverse reaction to the eucalyptus oil, wash it off immediately, and if you start to feel unwell, see your doctor.

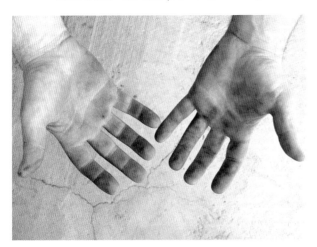

CAUTION: If you haven't used eucalyptus oil before – or haven't done so for a long time – you should do a skin patch test first (see page 96).

Hair

Hair Growth

Eucalyptus oil has many fans who use it for a variety of purposes including, in some cases, promoting hair growth. Add a few drops to your normal shampoo and massage your scalp while you wash your hair to help improve the flow of blood in your scalp to your hair roots. Wash the shampoo off as normal.

Some people rub neat eucalyptus on to their scalp at night and wash it off the next morning. Do be careful about trying this method, though. While some people use neat essential oil on their skin, many reliable sources say that you should not do this. Full-strength eucalyptus oil can be toxic and so should always be diluted before you put it on your skin. You should also always do a patch test on the skin of your forearm first and ask your doctor's advice if you are on any medications or suffer from the conditions mentioned above.

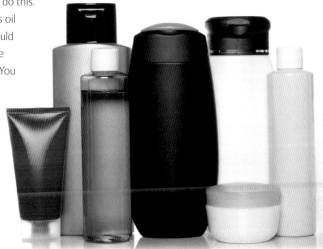

Shiny Hair

A glorious head of glossy hair is always a great confidence booster. Try this recipe for shiny locks. Pour out 50 ml/2 fl oz/¼ cup olive oil and 1 teaspoon eucalyptus oil, and mix them together. Massage the mixed oils into your scalp and comb through your hair (this will help stimulate the flow of blood to your roots). Put your hair in a clean towel, or a shower cap, and wait for 15–20 minutes. Then shampoo and condition your hair as usual.

You may find you need to shampoo more than once in order to get all the oil out. If you have a reaction to the oils – itching, for instance – wash them out of your hair at once. In order to make it easier to massage the oils into your scalp, once mixed, put them in a strong glass bottle and stand it in hot water for 5–10 minutes.

Itchy Scalp

If an itchy scalp is making life uncomfortable, you may be able to ease the problem with a home–made solution. Mix 50 ml/2 fl oz/ ¼ cup white vinegar with 1 teaspoon eucalyptus oil and 1 litre/1¾ pints/4 cups water. Put them in a container and shake well to mix them together. Bending over the bath or sink, rinse your hair with this a number of times, making sure your whole scalp has been covered. Then wash and condition your hair as you would normally. Before doing this, carry out a skin patch test (see page 96).

There are a number of different reasons why you might have an itchy scalp. For instance, it could be associated with dandruff or seborrhoeic dermatitis, whose symptoms include scaly and itchy skin on the scalp, face, ears, armpits and other areas. See your GP if you think you may have this condition.

Head Lice

These little creatures are an uncomfortable nuisance that can be hard to get rid of. They seem to spread in the blink of an eye, from one child to another and then to their siblings and parents, bringing an itchy scalp to all their hosts. Eucalyptus essential oil has been used for some time to combat head lice. Measure out a few drops of eucalyptus oil and mix it into 2 tablespoons of your normal shampoo. Use this solution to wash your child's (or your own) hair and cover with a shower cap for about 10 minutes (adults only).

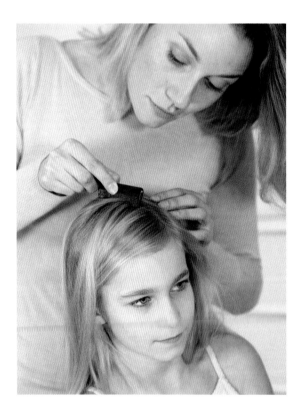

When the time is up (or straight away in the case of children) take the shower cap off, rinse the shampoo off and condition as normal. Combing the hair with a nit comb will help to remove lice and their eggs.

CAUTION: Do not use eucalyptus oil on or near babies and children aged two years and under, and always carry out a patch test before using even a weak solution on older children's hair. Also be extremely cautious in your use of eucalyptus oil on or near children aged two and over. Never allow children to swallow eucalyptus oil or anything containing it, as this can be dangerous to them.

Wellbeing

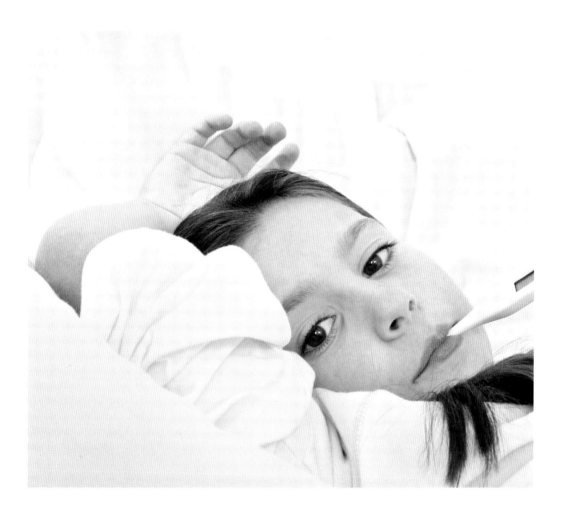

Stress Headaches

Eucalyptus oil can also be useful in relieving that common but painful problem of stress headaches. In a small study carried out in Europe, scientists tested volunteers to find out whether a mixture of peppermint oil, eucalyptus oil and ethanol (alcohol) could help to relieve this type of headache. The scientists discovered that this combination of oils and alcohol had a muscle-relaxing and mentally relaxing effect, which should help to relieve tension. The same study also found that this mixture increased cognitive performance (*see* opposite).

Boost Immune System

Among its health benefits, eucalyptus oil has the ability to kick-start a particular type of cell in our bodies. These cells are known as monocyte derived macrophages (MDMs), and they carry out a vital task, which is to fight infections. The effect eucalyptus oil has on MDMs is to trigger them into fighting mode, where they attack

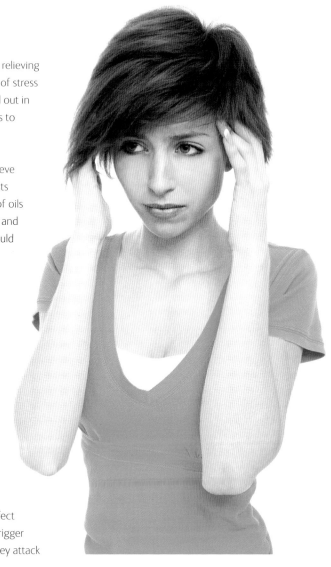

bacteria and other harmful substances. When the MDMs are in this state, they are known as phagocytes, and the way they behave is called the phagocytic response. The really important but simple message to remember about this process is that eucalyptus gives our immune system a helping hand.

Concentration and Alertness

Due to its invigorating smell, and its ability to help relieve sinus and congestion problems, eucalyptus oil is associated by some with a greater ability to concentrate and greater alertness. If you would like to try this yourself, simply put a few drops of eucalyptus on a ball of cotton wool or something similar. Then place the cotton wool out of reach of small children and animals, but close enough to allow you to breathe it in.

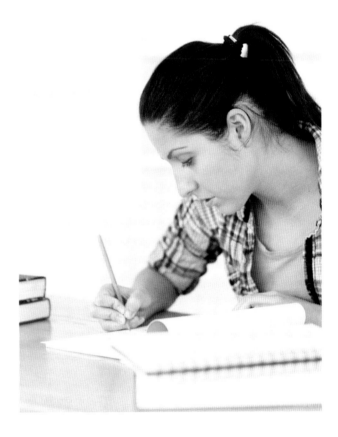

Alternatively, you could use eucalyptus oil in an aromatherapy diffuser, which warms the oil, releasing its vapour into your home.

Ailments
& Conditions

Keeping yourself and your family as healthy as possible can cover a wide range of skills and knowledge, from the simplest things, such as knowing how to sooth a sore throat or to remove a bee sting efficiently, to staying one step ahead when it comes to allergies and long-term conditions. Eucalyptus can give you a helping hand in different ways, ranging from keeping dust mites at bay to easing the pain of a sinus headache and making breathing easier when you have a cold.

Skin & Nails

CAUTION: See A Word of Warning on page 95 for important notes on when to avoid using eucalyptus.

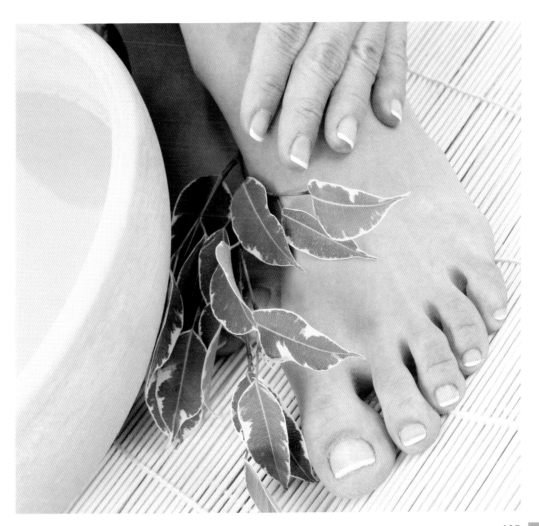

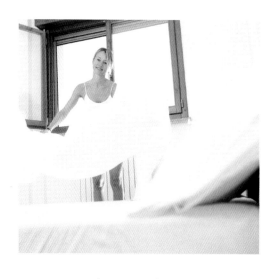

Eczema

Eczema, or dermatitis, as it's also known, is a long-term condition that can cause swollen, red and itchy skin. Atopic dermatitis is the most common version of this condition. It mostly affects babies and children and is an allergic condition, which means that it can be set off by contact with the things you are allergic to.

Dust mites are a common trigger for atopic dermatitis. One of their favourite places is your bed. A good way of keeping atopic dermatitis under control is to reduce your child's contact with dust mite allergens – and the bed is a good place to start. Experts advise putting a micro-porous cover on the mattress. This will seal mites in and stop new ones getting in. You can also put micro-porous covers on duvets and pillows, and put a cotton quilted cover over the mattress to absorb perspiration. You should also hot-wash all the bed linen every week.

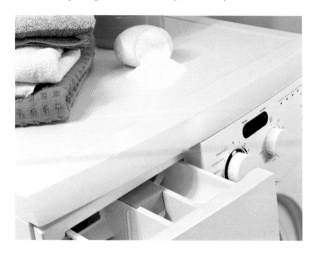

One way of improving your dust mite-busting technique is to add eucalyptus oil to your wash. About 25 drops in each load, along with your normal washing liquid or powder, should help keep dust mites at bay.

CAUTION: Eucalyptus can be an allergen for some people with eczema or dermatitis. If this is the case for your family, don't use it. You may want to ask your doctor before you try it out, as you don't want to cause an unnecessary flare-up of this condition.

Burns

Minor burns – the type that you can get from putting your skin in brief contact with a hot surface, such as the wire rack in a hot oven – can usually be dealt with at home. This type of

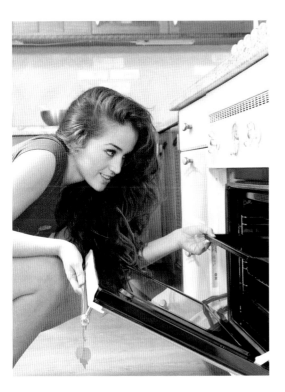

burn normally only affects the outer layer of the skin, causing some redness and pain, and they generally heal within several days to a week. If your burn is larger than a postage stamp, or deep, you should seek medical attention.

In the case of minor burns, carry out normal first-aid treatment: hold the burnt area under cold water for 10 minutes or until it becomes less painful. Then remove all jewellery and clothing from the affected area and cover the burn with a clean, non-fluffy material. Kitchen film, a clean plastic bag or clean cloth are all suitable. Some people use solutions including eucalyptus leaves or eucalyptus ointment to treat burns, as eucalyptus has antiflammatory and antiseptic properties, but it is advisable to talk to a pharmacist or your doctor before doing this.

Sunburn Relief

Spending too long in the sun without adequate protection – cover-up clothes and/or protective sun cream – can leave you with the inevitable sunburn and sore skin. If your sunburn is mild you can cool your skin down by putting a cold flannel over the burnt area, or by having a refreshing shower or bath. You should also drink plenty of water, which will help to replace fluid you may have lost and cool you down.

Calamine lotion may also help to relieve any itching and soreness, and lotions containing aloe vera should soothe the sore area. Some people use solutions including eucalyptus leaves or diluted eucalyptus oil to treat minor sunburns, but you must talk to a pharmacist or your doctor before doing this.

If you have more serious sunburn, feel faint or dehydrated, or have blisters, see your pharmacist or GP. You may require a cream specially designed for burns, and you may need to have dressings put on by a doctor or nurse. If a baby or child has been sunburned you should take them to your doctor.

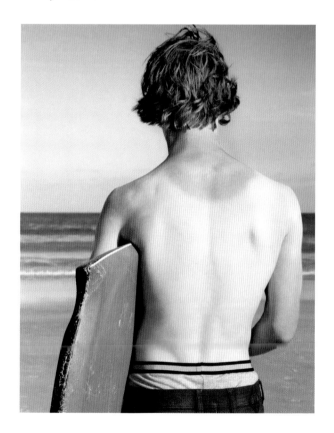

Insect Bites

Whether you're walking in the countryside, working in your garden, or indoors, you're nearly always vulnerable to insect bites. In many countries most of these don't cause a problem. However, if you have an allergic reaction to a bite or a sting you may need to get urgent medical attention. If you, or a child, scratch a bite, it can become infected and may start swelling or developing into a rash. In this case too, you would probably need to see a doctor.

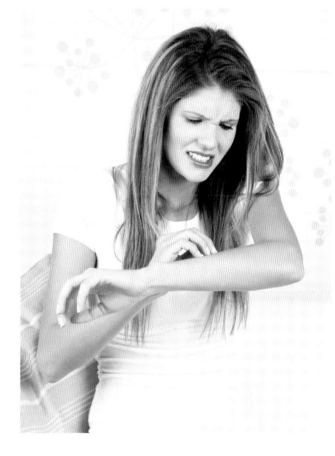

There are various creams that you can buy from your pharmacy and apply to relieve the pain and itching of an insect bite. Some people, though, dab diluted eucalyptus oil on bites. A well-stirred mixture of 8 drops of eucalyptus oil in 100 ml/3½ fl oz/⅓ cup water may help (do not use it at full strength). However, using eucalyptus oil before the mozzies and other biting insects appear may save you from being bitten at all. Eucalyptus oil has been used in insect repellents; also, some studies have shown that cineole, which comes from eucalyptus, repels mosquito bites.

Athlete's Foot

This fungal infection, also known as *tinea pedis*, can be a reminder that it may be time to rethink your footwear. It is closely related to ringworm (another fungal infection) and thrives in tight footwear that presses your toes together, damp socks and shoes, and warm, humid conditions. The signs to watch out for include itching, stinging and burning between the toes and on the soles of the feet, thick and crumbly toenails, and cracking and peeling skin between the toes and on the soles of the feet. Athlete's foot is contagious, so be careful about surfaces that could be contaminated, such as floors, and shoes, which may need to be thrown away.

If caught early enough, you can treat athlete's foot with antifungal medicines from your pharmacist. However, if you have diabetes, or have a fever or swollen feet, you should see your doctor (diabetics should go to their doctor as soon as they suspect they might have athlete's foot).

There are websites that suggest that eucalyptus may be useful for treating athlete's foot, and a study found that eucalyptus extract, with its antibacterial and antifungal properties, was effective against the pathogens that cause athlete's foot and other conditions. You should discuss with your doctor using some diluted eucalyptus oil to help.

Nail Fungal Infections

These unsightly infections can be tricky to tackle, and it can take some time before your nails are back to normal, but eucalyptus can help aid recovery. As a first step, you should see your doctor. Depending on the circumstances, they may decide to give you oral medication (medicine that you swallow) – if your nail is painful, for instance, or if you have diabetes. Another possibility is that your doctor may prescribe a topical medication – this means a cream or lotion that you paint on to your affected nails.

There are steps that you can and should take to help rid yourself of a fungal infection and to prevent it returning. Keep your feet as clean, cool and dry as possible. Make sure your nails are always cut short, and keep a separate set of nail clippers to use only on the infected nails. Throw away old, worn shoes and, if you have to wear socks, choose cotton ones. Also, try to wear trainers as little as possible.

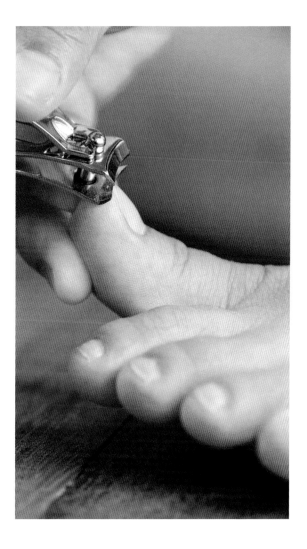

Eucalyptus to the Rescue

Thanks to its antibacterial and antifungal properties, eucalyptus oil may be able to help deal with nail fungal infections. If your doctor agrees that it is safe to try this at home (see below), ask them to suggest a suitable dilution – for instance, a few drops of eucalyptus oil in 100 ml/3½ fl oz/⅓ cup water. Then paint this mixture on to the affected nail using a cotton bud. Before you do this, carry out a patch test on your inner forearm and leave it for 24 hours to see if you have an adverse reaction.

Another treatment that has had positive feedback is using a shop–bought vapour rub which contains eucalyptus oil and other substances. As this is purely anecdotal, there is no scientific proof that it works (again, see below) and no suggested dosage.

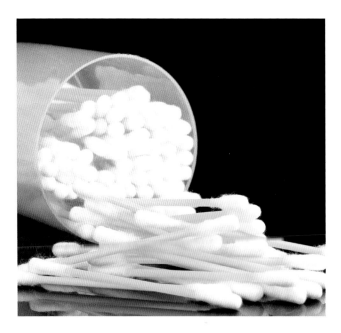

CAUTION: Always speak to your doctor before using eucalyptus oil, in any form, to treat nail fungal infections. Your doctor will want to make sure that it is safe for you to do this by checking on any existing medical conditions you have and also by checking on whether eucalyptus oil is likely to affect any medicine you are taking for other conditions.

Chest & Throat

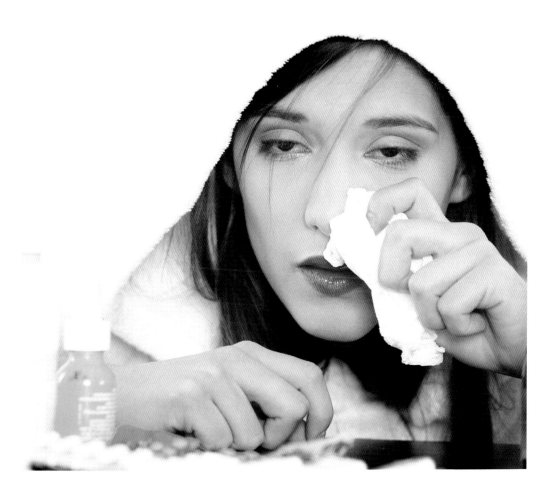

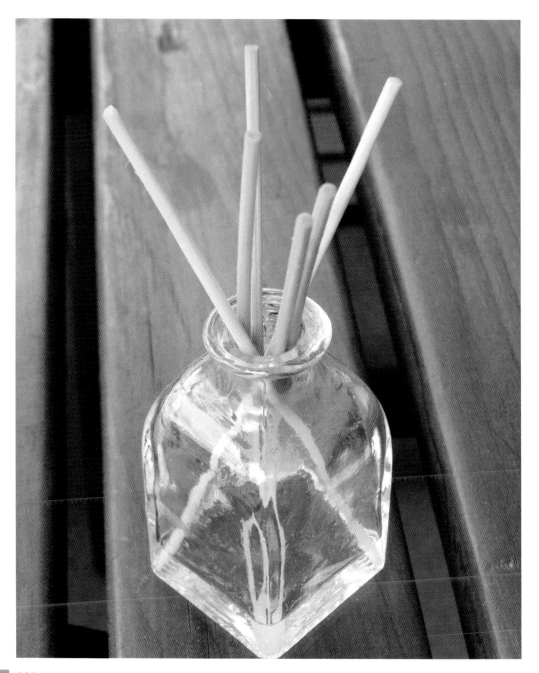

Decongestant

That stuffed-up, bunged-up feeling that we get in our noses may be one of the worst aspects of having a cold. Not only can it make us sound funny – to other people, at least – it can also be uncomfortable, even painful, and prevent us from breathing through our noses and hearing properly. As shown in a scientific study, eucalyptus oil can help to relieve the discomfort and feeling of pressure by acting as a decongestant. There are different ways in which you can use eucalyptus oil in this situation.

You can put a few drops of the oil on a tissue, or cotton wool ball, and place it near you, but out of the reach of small children. You could also buy an ointment or rub that includes eucalyptus as an ingredient and rub this on your chest or back. Eucalyptus oil can help to loosen phlegm – the rather unpleasant, thick mucus that you get in your airways when you have an infection – and to make you feel more comfortable.

Freshen Up

If you've been sick for a while, you can start to feel the presence of those germs all around you! You can deodorize a sick room by using some eucalyptus oil in a diffuser or vaporizer, which will heat the oil and release the vapour into the air. This will not only freshen the room but should help with the symptoms of a cold or congestion too. It may also make breathing easier as you try to sleep.

Colds

Colds can sneak up on us at any time of year, leaving us with a stuffy and runny nose, sore throat, cough and sneezing. There are more than 200 viruses that can cause colds, which explains why when you've just got rid of one cold you catch another. Colds usually get better by themselves. If you, or anyone in your family, have a cold you can take basic steps to treat

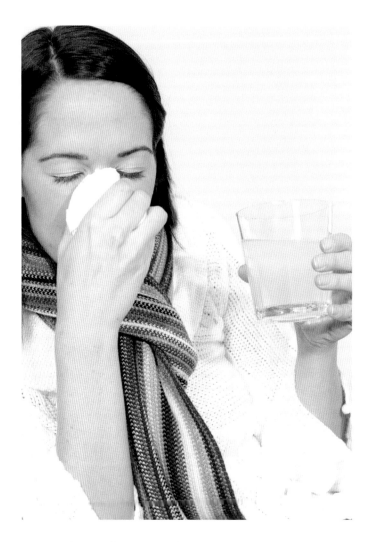

the symptoms and make life a little more comfortable. First of all, make sure that you drink plenty of fluids to keep yourself properly hydrated. Also, take it easy and get plenty of rest until you feel well again, and don't forget to eat healthy food – including five portions of fruit and vegetables a day.

One great way for some relief is to make yourself a bath with a few essential oils added in to help relieve the symptoms of a cold. Add 3 drops eucalyptus oil, 3 drops lavender oil and 2 drops mint oil to a carrier oil and then add the solution to your bath and relax!

CAUTION: Do not be tempted to keep adding more oil, as less is more, and you don't want to risk irritating your skin with an excess of essential oil.

Steam Inhalation

There is a simple way of easing your congestion: steam inhalation. Get a heatproof bowl and pour hot water into it. Add a few drops of eucalyptus oil and then lean forward with a towel draped over your head. The towel will help to trap the vapours, and the steam and eucalyptus should help to clear your nose and make it easier to breathe clearly. You can also try putting a few drops of eucalyptus oil on a cotton wool ball or clean cloth, and leaving it in the bathroom while you shower or bath. Alternatively, put a few drops on a clean handkerchief and breathe the vapour when you need to.

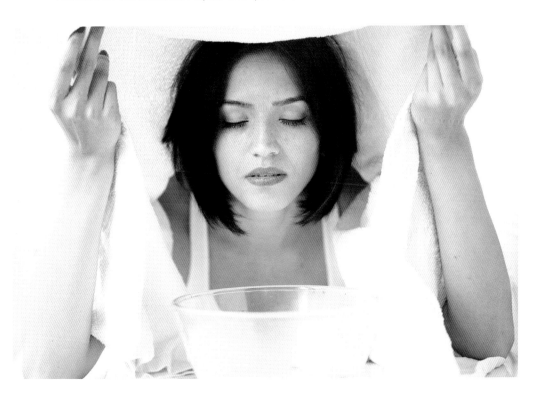

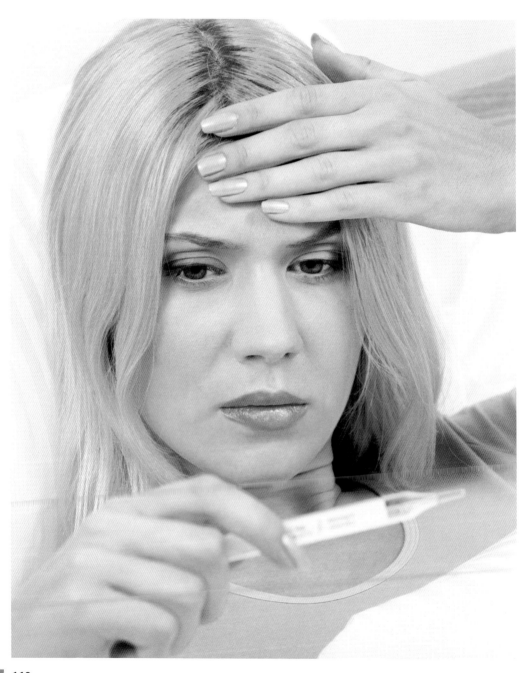

Flu Symptoms

This viral illness is quite different from a cold.
It's caused by different viruses and seems to hit
you out of the blue, with more extreme
symptoms than you'd have with a cold. The bad
news is that it can last for longer. One of the
first signs that you have flu (short for influenza)
is the sudden arrival of a number of symptoms,
including aches and pains, a headache, high
temperature, sore throat and feeling tired.

This unwelcome mixture of symptoms can
make you feel quite unwell and send you to
your bed. Most normally healthy people don't
need to see a doctor when they have flu, but if
you have a long-term medical condition, such
as heart disease, are over 65 or pregnant you
may need to see your doctor.

Flu Relief

Self-help steps that you can take to make
yourself feel more comfortable include drinking
plenty of water, taking paracetamol or
ibuprofen (but be careful not to overdose) and
resting. A few drops of eucalyptus oil on a
cotton wool ball, placed in your bedroom and
other rooms in the house, may help you to
breathe more easily.

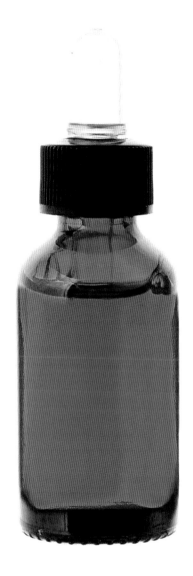

Sinus Infections

If you have ever suffered with sinusitis (also known as rhinosinusitis), you will know how miserable it can make you feel. This condition is triggered when the lining of your sinuses – the cavities in both cheeks, between your eyes and above your eye sockets – become swollen due to infection. The result is facial pain near the sinuses, which may become worse when you move your head, a blocked or runny nose, a headache, tiredness and feeling pretty unwell. In most cases you won't need to see your doctor, but there are steps you can take to help yourself feel better If your symptoms don't improve after a week, are getting worse or keep coming back, see your doctor..

A study of about 300 people found that using eucalyptus oil along with two other essential oils – d–limonene and alpha–pinene – improved the symptoms of acute sinusitis.

Rest if you can, sleeping with your head raised, and drink plenty of fluids. Steaming your nasal cavities may also help, although it may only be a temporary break from that blocked nose. Pour hot water into a heatproof bowl, add a couple of drops of eucalyptus oil to it and then lean forward over the bowl so that you can breathe in the steam rising up. Draping a towel over your head and the bowl of hot water should make this more effective, as it will help to trap the steam.

CAUTION: Eucalyptus oil, used as an inhalant and around the house, can be beneficial to people with asthma. However, it can also act as a trigger for asthma attacks, so always use with caution and check with your doctor. If eucalyptus oil triggers an episode of asthma, stop using it.

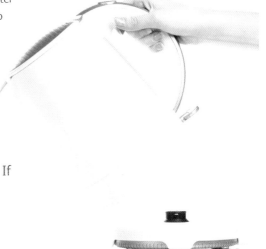

Bronchitis Explained

If you have acute bronchitis – a lung infection – it should clear up within a few weeks, and you may not need to see your doctor about it (unless you have other underlying conditions; see below). The main symptom of bronchitis is a cough, which can bring up mucus of a yellow–grey colour. You may also feel wheezy and experience tightness across your chest, with a slight fever and general aches and pains.

If your cough is very bad and goes on for more than three weeks, the mucus you're coughing up is streaked with blood and you become drowsy, you should see your doctor straight away. In some cases, bronchitis symptoms can be similar to those of pneumonia – coughing, high temperature and trouble breathing – so you do need to be careful and watch out for any worsening of your condition.

CAUTION: If you have asthma, emphysema, congestive heart failure or any other condition that affects your heart or lungs, see your doctor.

Eucalyptus for Bronchitis

A number of studies have been carried out into whether eucalyptus oil (combined with two related oils and known collectively as Essential Oil Monoterpenes) can help with acute and chronic bronchitis, and sinus infections. One study on 676 people with acute bronchitis found that two weeks of treatment with Essential Oil Monoterpenes was as effective as taking antibiotics for reducing symptoms and helping recovery. The study used a specially made medicine that was swallowed by the patients, as eucalyptus oil on its own is toxic and must never be swallowed in undiluted form. Even diluted eucalyptus oil must not be taken without advice from your doctor.

However, eucalyptus oil may be able to help you feel more comfortable. Put a few drops on a tissue or cotton wool ball and place this in your bedroom and wherever else you spend most time around the house (but make sure it is out if the reach of children). A steam inhalation may also help: add a couple of drops of eucalyptus oil to a bowl of hot water, drape a towel over your head to catch the steam and put your head over the bowl. This may help ease your symptoms. Everyone is different, though, so if having eucalyptus oil near you makes you cough, stop using it.

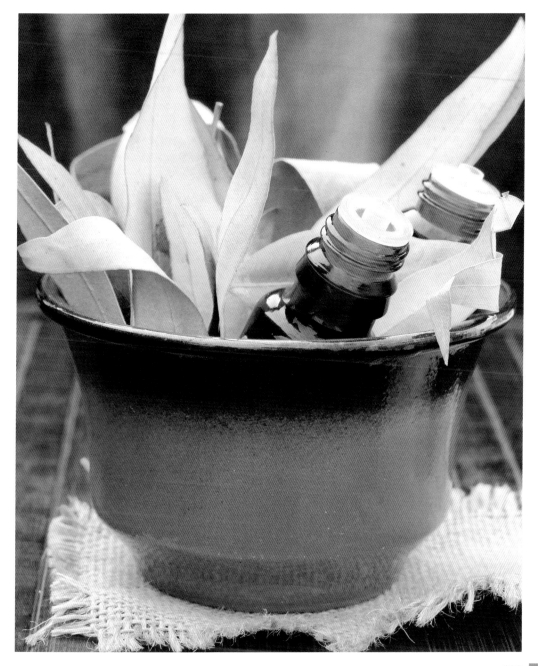

That Nasty Cough

Eucalyptus can help bring blissful relief to that cough that just won't go away. The most common cause of a cough is a respiratory tract infection. This will have been caused by a virus that has in turn caused the cold, flu or bronchitis. Coughs can take different forms: they can be dry, tickly and non–productive (they don't produce mucus) or chesty. The latter are productive – you often cough up phlegm, or thick mucus, from your airways. As unpleasant as this sounds, it is actually a good thing, because it can help ease your coughing.

Your cough should disappear once the viral infection that caused it has gone. If your cough doesn't clear up in two weeks' time, or is getting steadily worse, you should see your GP. If you have a child with a cough there are important signs to watch out for. These include: a cough that doesn't get better or gets worse, coughing when eating or feeding, coughing that keeps bringing up phlegm, and a child who has night sweats or is losing weight. These symptoms may be a sign that your child has something more serious than just a cough, and you should take them to your GP straight away.

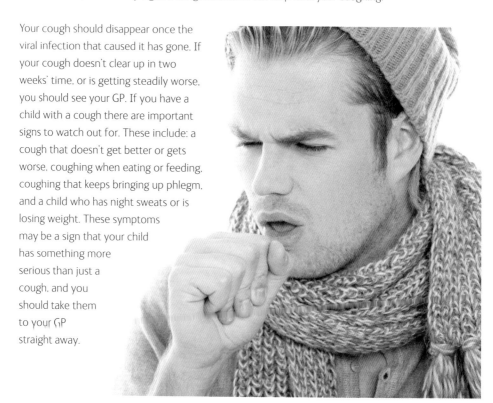

Cough Relief

Eucalyptus is a common ingredient in lots of over-the-counter medicine to treat coughs and colds. You'll find it in the ingredients list of pastilles, lozenges and vapour rubs. Eucalyptus oil has been found to help loosen phlegm or mucus, and that in turn can help to ease a cough. You can put a few drops on a tissue, piece of cloth or cotton wool buds, and place them in your bedroom, bathroom or nearby when

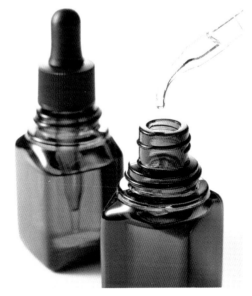

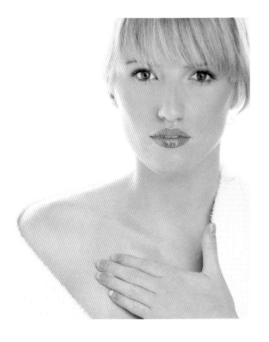

you are resting (make sure that you put them out of the reach of children, though).

Unless you have had a bad reaction to eucalyptus at any time, you can apply a vapour rub. Doing this before going to sleep can help you have a better night's rest. One suggested recipe for making your own vapour rub is to put 6 drops of eucalyptus oil in 1 tablespoon base oil, such as olive or sunflower oil. Do a skin patch test first (*see* page 96) and do not use on young children without checking with your doctor first.

Aches & Pains

Massage Oil

There are many different types of massage oil available in the shops and online, so you can choose from a huge range of ready-made options. However, you can also easily make your own. There are two basic factors involved in the making of massage oil. The base or carrier oil is the one that you'll need most of. As its name suggests, this is the base for the essential oil or oils that will add their particular properties and scents to the finished massage oil. Popular base or carrier oils are sweet almond, grape seed, jojoba oil and olive oil.

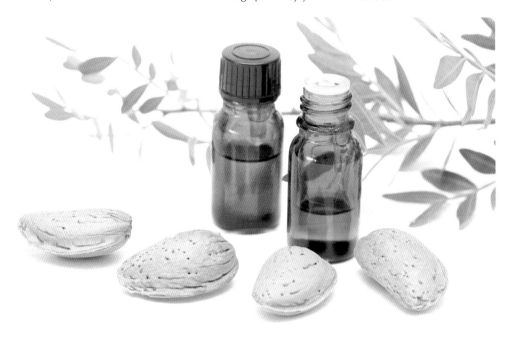

There is also a wide range of essential oils to select from. Eucalyptus essential oil, with its antiseptic, disinfectant and decongestant properties, is a good choice for helping with colds, flu, sinusitis and other conditions. You can, if you wish, add some other complementary oils, but you do have to check first that they do fit with eucalyptus and are suitable for the purpose. A recipe for cold relief massage oil, for instance, includes 5 drops each of eucalyptus, lavender oil, peppermint oil and tea tree oil in 120 ml/4 fl oz/½ cup carrier oil. In order to create a home-made muscle rub, use about 10 drops of eucalyptus oil in around 50 ml/2 fl oz/¼ cup carrier oil.

CAUTION: Do a skin patch test before you use the massage oil. If you have an extreme reaction, see your doctor. If you don't have a reaction then the massage oil should be safe to use.

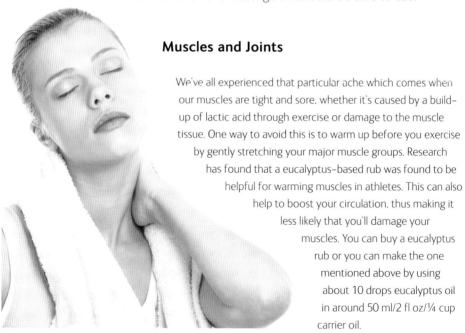

Muscles and Joints

We've all experienced that particular ache which comes when our muscles are tight and sore, whether it's caused by a build-up of lactic acid through exercise or damage to the muscle tissue. One way to avoid this is to warm up before you exercise by gently stretching your major muscle groups. Research has found that a eucalyptus-based rub was found to be helpful for warming muscles in athletes. This can also help to boost your circulation, thus making it less likely that you'll damage your muscles. You can buy a eucalyptus rub or you can make the one mentioned above by using about 10 drops eucalyptus oil in around 50 ml/2 fl oz/¼ cup carrier oil.

Just Relax

A nice hot bath can do wonders for relaxation, but adding a bit of eucalyptus oil can really help those aches and pains. Add 4 drops eucalyptus oil, 3 drops thyme oil and 3 drops clary sage oil to a carrier oil, and then pour the solution into your bath and wash the pain away.

Arthritis Relief

There are a number of different types of arthritis, but one of the most common is osteoarthritis. In this condition the cartilage between the bones gradually disintegrates, so the bones rub against each other, which causes pain and inflammation in and around the joints. Not surprisingly, this can mean that people with arthritis find that their movement is restricted, their joints are stiff and, as a consequence, their muscles start losing strength and become weaker.

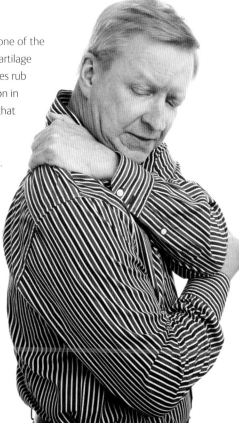

If you have osteoarthritis your doctor may prescribe medication to help ease the discomfort. There are a number of treatments for osteoarthritis, including painkillers, non-steroidal anti-inflammatory drugs and corticosteroids. Eucalyptus can help to soothe the pain that comes with osteoarthritis. Cineole, which is the active component in eucalyptus oil, helps the nerves around the blood vessels to relax. This helps to improve circulation, which in turn helps to reduce the pain and inflammation. Do not use any eucalyptus products, or eucalyptus rubs or bath salts, without your doctor's approval.

Sore Feet Massage

Treat yourself – or someone else – to a quick, soothing foot rub after a tiring day. Mix together 120 ml/4 fl oz/½ cup olive or sweet almond oil and ½ teaspoon eucalyptus oil. Warm the oils by rubbing the mixture between your hands and gently massage your feet. Make sure you have a clean pair of cotton socks at hand to put on once the massage is over.

Eucalyptus oil and products are usually safe, if they are properly diluted and you follow reliable instructions. However, you should not give it to children aged two and under, and you should seek medical advice before using it on or near children aged 12 and under. You need to take particular care if you have a long–standing illness, such as asthma or epilepsy. Again, check with your doctor or pharmacist before use.

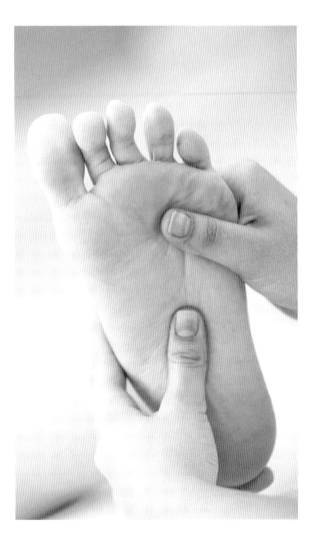

CAUTION: If you are pregnant, breastfeeding, or have severe liver or kidney disease, the general advice is not to use eucalyptus oil.

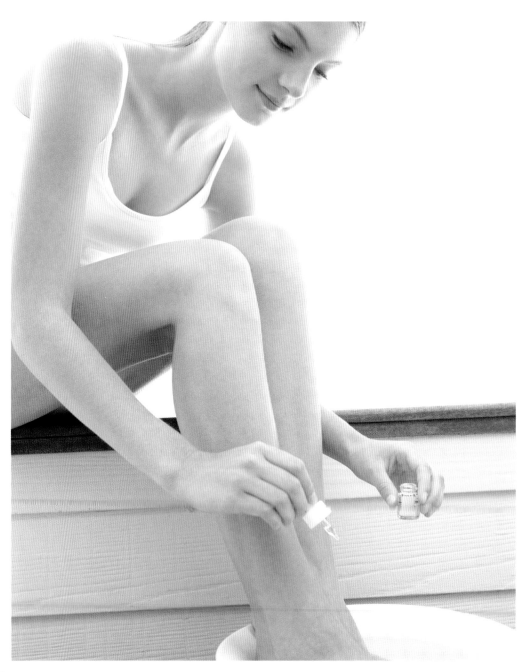

Aching Feet Foot Bath

If you've been on your feet all day, especially when you're not in comfortable shoes, your feet may well be aching by the time you get home. Rather than putting your feet up (if you get a chance), give your feet a treat with a soothing foot bath. Find a clean bowl or container that is large enough for you to put both feet into comfortably. Pour warm (but not too hot) water into the bowl and add 1 teaspoon eucalyptus oil. Give your feet a decent soak, allowing yourself at least 10 minutes.

Once you have finished, dry your feet vigorously with a towel. If you feel like it, you can follow the foot bath with a foot massage. Simply massage your feet with your usual foot lotion, put on clean cotton socks and put your feet up.

Backache

The onset of backache can really ruin your day, and can be brought on by such things as having to do a lot of heavy lifting. Make yourself a eucalyptus hot compress to soothe your back. Heat 100 ml/3½ fl oz/⅓ cup water in a saucepan and heat. When very hot, add 5 drops eucalyptus oil and cover. After a couple of minutes, using rubber gloves, uncover the pan, and lay a flannel over the water to absorb some of it. Squeeze out any excess water and then place against your back. When the flannel cools, reheat.

CAUTION: Test the compress is not too hot on a small area of skin before applying fully to your back.

Stiff Neck

The stresses of the day can cause your neck to develop that familiar ache. Ease the pain with a hot compress infused with eucalyptus oil (*see* Backache) to soothe those sore muscles.

Oral Remedies

Mouthwash

Are you a regular rinser? Or perhaps you can't see the point of mouthwash?

One leading American hospital says on its website that mouthwash can help to prevent plaque build-up on teeth and gums, and that it controls gingivitis (see below) and bad breath. You do need to take care when you use mouthwash: you should hold it in your mouth and swish it around for about 30 seconds and then spit it out. You should not swallow mouthwash. Some brands contain alcohol, which is one reason why it is especially important to spit the mouthwash out.

CAUTION: Do not put undiluted eucalyptus oil in your mouth or swallow it. You should take your doctor's advice before swallowing any product or mixture containing eucalyptus oil. It can be particularly dangerous for children, so do not leave it, or any products containing eucalyptus oil, anywhere near kids.

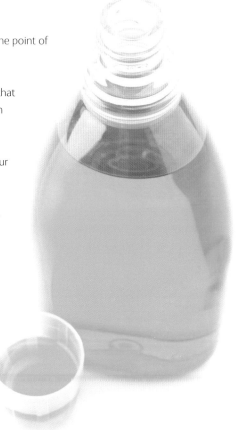

Eucalyptus oil can be found in a number of branded mouthwashes, which are likely to be safe for most healthy people to use, as long as the instructions are followed. Eucalyptus and other oils are used in some antiseptic mouthwashes and these have been shown to help prevent plaque and gingivitis. Do make sure that you follow the instructions for frequency of use and correct amounts on each occasion. In order to make your own mouthwash, add a few drops of eucalyptus oil to a large glass of water. Rinse your mouth and then spit the water/oil mixture out. Do not give to children. If you have an adverse reaction, see your doctor.

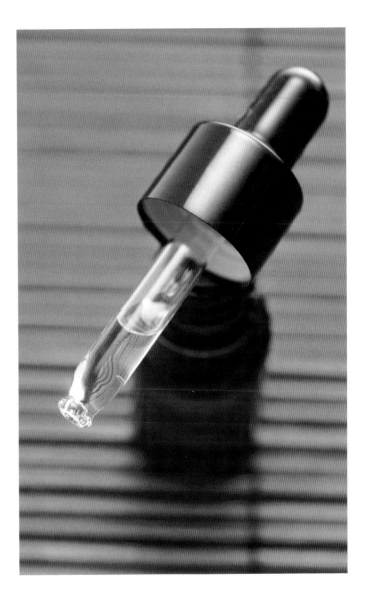

Mouth Ulcers

Mouth ulcers are extremely common. Most of us will experience them during our lifetime, and they usually clear up on their own. They can be caused by accidentally biting the inside of your mouth or by a sharp tooth. Some people find that they suffer from recurrent ulcers, which just keep coming back. These can be caused by stress, hormone changes during your period, certain foods or because this is a trait passed on through their family. Ulcers can also be caused by medical conditions, including lack of iron, coeliac disease, irritable bowel disease, chickenpox and vitamin B12 deficiency.

To ease the discomfort, use a soft toothbrush, eat soft, easy-to-chew foods and reduce your stress levels if you can. It's important to keep on cleaning and flossing your teeth thoroughly every day. Ask your pharmacist for advice on suitable medication. They may suggest an antimicrobial mouthwash, which can help in the fight against bacteria and viruses, or corticosteroids in order to bring down the inflammation. You may need to see your GP to have this on prescription and they may also prescribe a painkiller in the form of a mouthwash or spray.

Gargling with a eucalyptus and water mouthwash may help to ease the discomfort of mouth ulcers. To make your own mouthwash, add a few drops of eucalyptus oil to a large glass of water. Rinse your mouth and then spit the water/oil mixture out. Do not swallow and do not give to children. If you have an adverse reaction, rinse your mouth out with water and do not use the eucalyptus mix again. However, if you have a severe adverse reaction, see your doctor straight away.

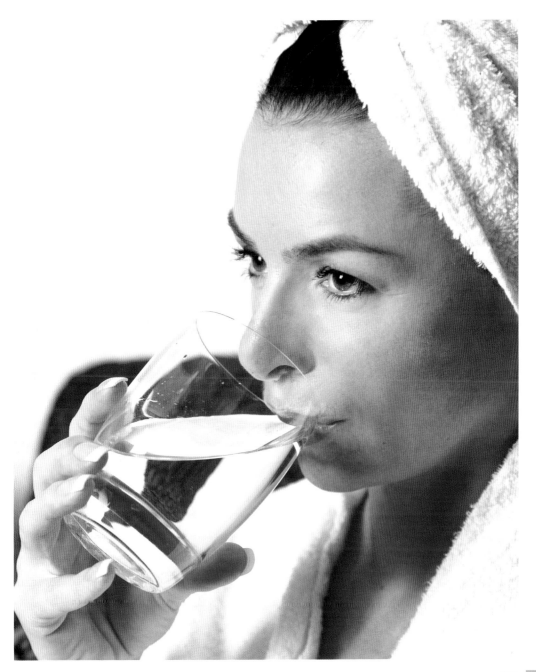

Plaque and Gingivitis

Gingivitis is one of the conditions (along with periodontitis) that come under the heading of gum disease. If you have gingivitis, the first symptoms you're likely to notice are red and swollen gums. You may also notice that your gums bleed after you've cleaned or flossed your teeth. However, you may not realise that you have gingivitis until you visit your dentist (which is why it's important to keep your regular dental appointments). If gingivitis isn't dealt with, it can develop into periodontitis, which can mean that your teeth become loose, and you may develop an abscess in your gums.

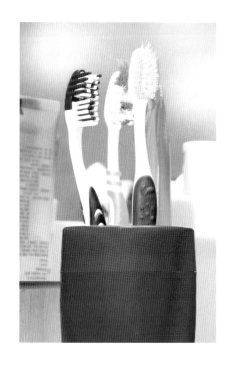

The usual treatment for gingivitis is to take better care of your teeth. Your dentist may refer to this as good oral hygiene, which means that you need to

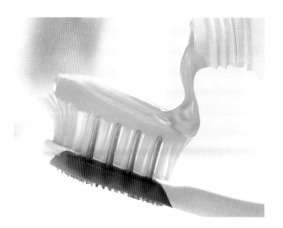

brush your teeth twice a day, making sure that you get to the back of all your teeth – including the ones at the back of your mouth. Your dentist will be able to show you the most effective way of brushing your teeth and may recommend using an electric toothbrush. Brushing with toothpaste containing fluoride and eucalyptus should help to keep decay at bay. You should also floss your teeth – every day if possible – and avoid smoking.

A study carried out in people who had gingivitis found that those who chewed gum containing eucalyptus saw improvements in their condition. These improvements included a reduction in bleeding from the gums and decreased amounts of plaque. The conclusion was that using gum or toothpaste containing eucalyptus extract could be good for your teeth and mouth.

Bad Breath

Bad breath can be a warning sign of gum disease. And the most common cause of bad breath is the same as that for gum disease: poor oral hygiene. It's interesting that one possible treatment for gum disease may also be helpful for treating bad breath (*see* Mouthwash on page 134). Mouthwash containing eucalyptus and other essential oils can be helpful in treating bad breath, but you also have to maintain good oral hygiene habits.

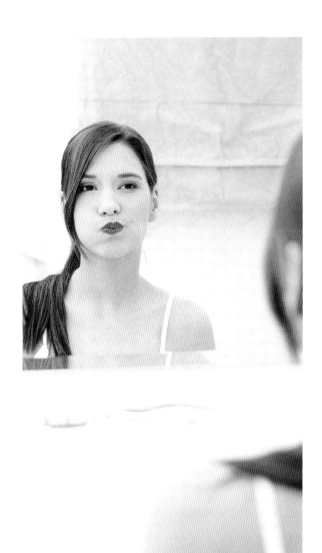

Outdoors & Maintenance

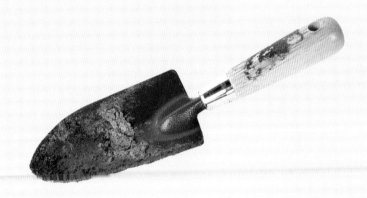

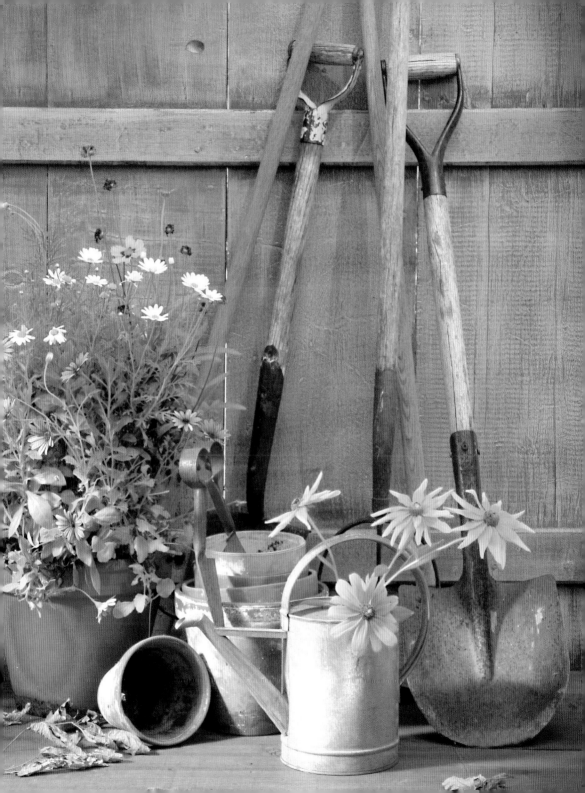

Garden

For many keen gardeners it's important to have the chance to tend plants and trees without adding harmful chemicals to the environment. The antiseptic and antibacterial properties of eucalyptus make it a useful tool for those who want to keep pests of all kinds off their plants – and away from themselves. Taking good care of tools and equipment is also a lesson that's learned early on in a gardener's training. The hints in this section show how eucalyptus oil can be used in simple ways to make the best of your garden.

Pests

Plant Spray

If you love your garden you'll
be aware of the constant
battle that gardeners have
with garden pests such as
aphids, whiteflies, earwigs and
snails. Make your own pest–
repelling spray using
1 teaspoon eucalyptus oil,
20 ml/¾ fl oz/1 ½ tbsp Canola
(or sunflower) oil, ⅓ tsp any
dishwashing detergent and
1 litre/2 pints/4 cups water.

Use this mixture
immediately, in a spray
bottle, on roses, azaleas,
cucumbers, tomatoes,
strawberries, and so on.
Then spray again, three to
five days later. If there are
a lot of insects in your
garden, make the mixture
more concentrated. After
using, wash the spray bottle
out thoroughly.

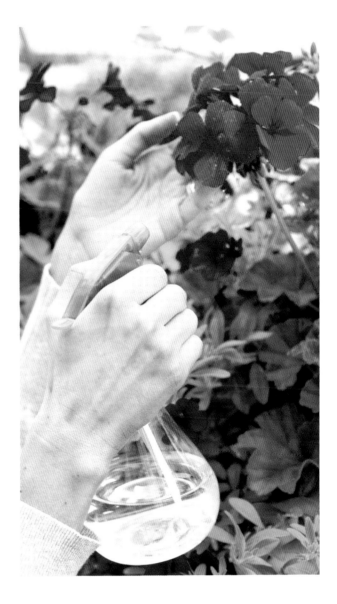

Insect Repellent for People

Of course, plants aren't the only things bothered by garden pests. Keep mosquitoes away with this easy-to-make insect repellent. Mix 100 ml/3 ½ fl oz/⅓ cup Canola (or sunflower or other unscented) oil with 30 drops of eucalyptus oil, and, if you like, 30 drops of citronella oil, which is especially useful in areas with particularly bad insect problems. Shake the liquids together in a bottle and then pour some into your hand. Apply to all exposed areas, as with any insect repellent.

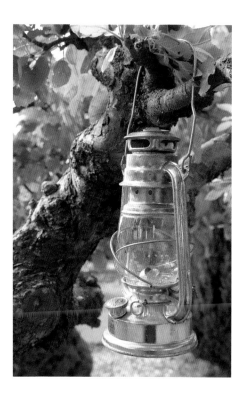

Garden Lamps

If you have lamps or lanterns around your garden that you light at night, turn them into insect repellents too. Simply mix some eucalyptus oil with the kerosene in the lamps and light them as usual.

Repelling Cats

Cats can cause havoc in a lovingly tended garden, hunting for young birds and using the soil as a toilet. Mix a solution of 2 teaspoons eucalyptus oil and 200 ml/7 fl oz/¾ cup water in a spray bottle and shake well. Squirt in all the places where you've previously seen cats clawing, scratching or going to the toilet. Don't forget paths, doorways and even the tops of fences – anywhere they might walk or climb up in order to get into your garden.

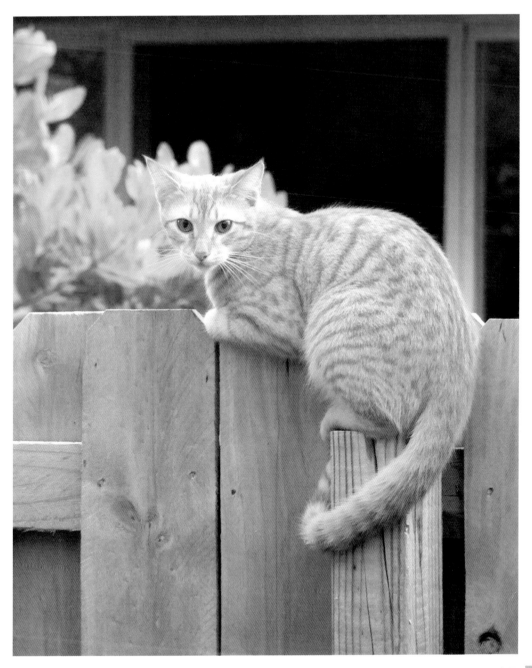

Cleaning

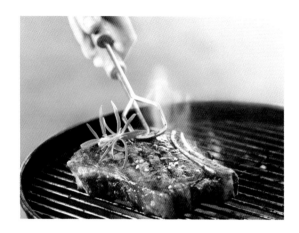

Degreasing Barbecues

Having to clean up the barbecue is always rather a letdown once the party's over. Tackle it with a bucketful of hot soapy water and 2 teaspoons eucalyptus oil. Wash the grease and burnt bits off the barbecue using a scrubbing brush or scouring pad and, once it's clean, rinse it – ready for the next time.

Washing Tools

Out in the garden, we use tools for a wide variety of jobs, such as cutting down or digging up diseased plants and planting new ones. In order to avoid infecting the new plants with harmful bacteria from the diseased ones, make sure you wash your tools in between tasks. Clean off the dirt and then wash them in hot water into which you have stirred 2 teaspoons eucalyptus oil. Leave the tools out to dry or wipe them dry before you put them away.

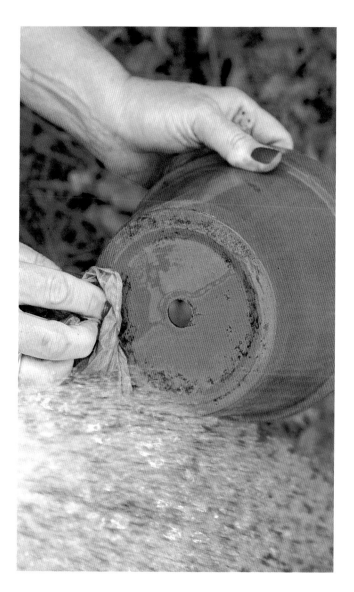

Washing Plant Pots

Plant pots can harbour bacteria and other nasties, so make sure you wash them thoroughly before you use them again. Get a bucketful of hot, soapy water, add 5 ml/⅙ fl oz/1 tsp eucalyptus oil and give the pots a good scrub. Then rinse them in clear water and leave to dry before you put them away or use them again.

Washing Paint Brushes

We're all guilty occasionally of neglecting our equipment. If you've been painting with oil paints and haven't cleaned the brushes properly, a good solution for getting them clean is to soak them in eucalyptus oil – a natural and much fresher–smelling alternative to turpentine.

Vehicles

Whether your car is your pride and joy or just a means of getting yourself and your family around and picking up the shopping, it's still important that it's a clean and hygienic vehicle in which to travel. Making your car a more pleasant place doesn't have to involve a lot of expense or time. In this section we look at quick and simple ways to disinfect and deodorize the interior, and we also describe how to spruce up the exterior – and even your parking space.

Odour

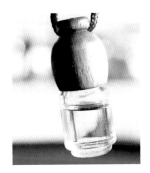

Deodorize Interiors

Cars have become so much a part of our lives that they are almost like an extra room. However, sometimes they can go a long time between spring-cleaning sessions. In order to get your car smelling good enough to travel in (with the windows closed), make up a eucalyptus spray by using 1 teaspoon eucalyptus oil for every 500 ml/18 fl oz/2 cups water. Pour this mixture into a spray bottle, shake and spray, and you'll instantly have a fresh-smelling interior.

Reinvigorate Air Fresheners

Car fresheners do run out of freshness eventually. Rather than buying a new one, put a few drops of eucalyptus oil on your existing freshener and enjoy that fresh car smell again.

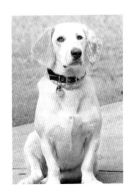

Stop Dogs Marking Tyres

Dogs urinate on things – among them bins, fences, posts, trees and tyres – to mark their territory and let other dogs know they've been there. You can try to train your dog not to wee on your tyres, but it's hard to do so with a neighbour's or friend's dog. Instead, use eucalyptus oil to put an unappealing smell on your car tyres by adding a few drops of it (you can always add more if it needs to smell stronger) to some water in a spray bottle and coating your tyres with the solution.

Cleaning

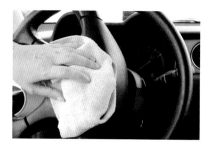

Car Interiors

Even car owners who are strict about not bringing food/muddy boots/pets into their treasured vehicle will want to clean their car effectively. And for those who are less strict, being able to clean, disinfect and deodorize their car in one go will be a time-saving boon. Make up a solution of 1 teaspoon eucalyptus oil for every 500 ml/18 fl oz/2 cups water and pour into a clean spray bottle. This, with a couple of clean cloths, is all the equipment you need to make your car thoroughly clean and disinfected.

Removing Sticky Marks

Sandwiches, drinks, sun cream ... The culprits behind those sticky marks on your dashboard, doors and upholstery are too many to name. Rather than letting them spoil your journey, get rid of them. Wipe them away with a few drops of eucalyptus oil on a clean cloth, or with a eucalyptus spray solution (1 teaspoon eucalyptus oil for every 500 ml/18 fl oz/2 cups water). Always remember to carry out a patch test first in a place where it won't be obvious.

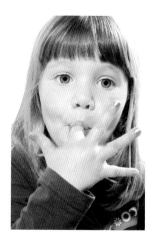

Other sticky marks are those left behind by stickers such as old bumper stickers you have peeled away because you no longer want them. Put a couple of drops eucalyptus oil on a cloth and wipe over the residue. Leave for a little while then wipe away

Removing Tar Marks from Paintwork

It's a habitual problem for car owners – how do you get tar off your paintwork? It doesn't have to be an expensive job, and you don't even have to go near a garage. Find a clean cloth and put on enough drops of eucalyptus oil to make the cloth feel damp. This should take the marks off. If you have a large area to tackle, mix up the following solution: one part eucalyptus oil and four parts of either petrol or vinegar. Make sure you rinse the affected paintwork once you have finished.

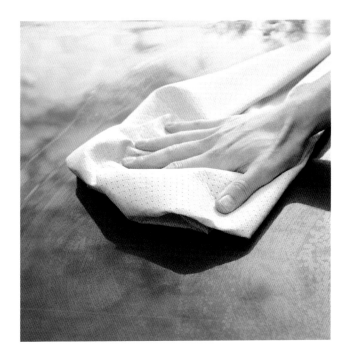

Cleaning Driveways and Garage Floors

A stained driveway or garage floor is never going to give you a warm welcome home. Tackle these unsightly stains with a bucketful of hot soapy water into which you have added 2 teaspoons eucalyptus oil before stirring. Get a sturdy scrubbing brush to clean the stain off. Once you're happy with the result, wash the soapy water off with clean water. If the stain is a new grease spillage, cover the damp patch with sawdust or cat litter, leave overnight and then carry on as above.

Growing Eucalyptus

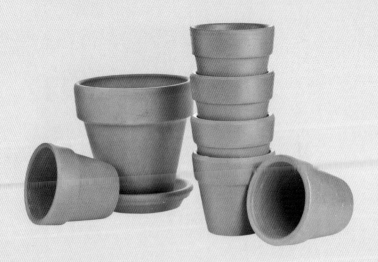

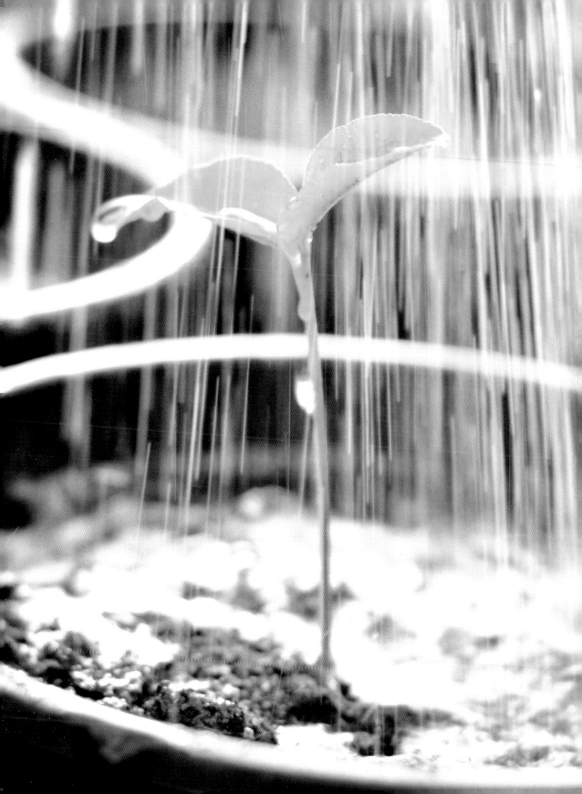

Preparing to Grow

The eucalyptus is a plant that we strongly associate with Australia – rather like the koalas that exist solely on its leaves. But the gumtree – as it's often affectionately known in its homeland – isn't only found down under. Its fragrant scent, delicately coloured silvery blue-green leaves and striking, multi-coloured bark have made it a favourite in gardens, parks and flower arrangements in countries around the world. With the benefit of a little gardening knowledge, it's possible to have a eucalyptus all of your own.

Tools

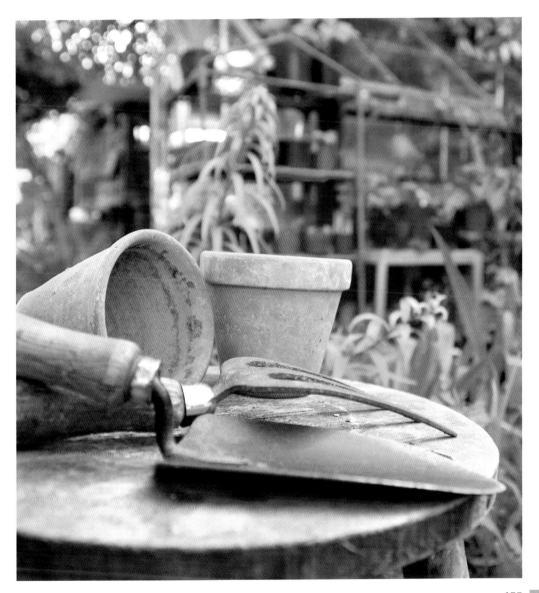

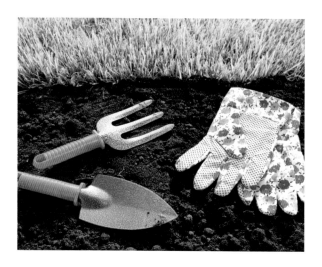

Choosing the Right Tools

Every task is easier if you have the right tools, and growing eucalyptus plants is no different from growing any other type of plant. Before you embark on any gardening job, make sure that you have all the tools you need laid out in front of you, so that you won't have to break off from what you're doing to hunt for something.

It's also important that your tools are clean, so that you don't pass bacteria and pest eggs or larvae on to your new plants (*see* pages 146–47 for tips on how eucalyptus oil can help keep your tools and plant pots). Remember that you may need different tools – for instance, different-sized plant pots – depending on the size of the plant.

Think about the task you want to carry out. Are you germinating your own plants from seeds or are you potting on seedlings? You won't need many tools for these tasks apart from clean containers: as many small ones as you have seeds, if you are planting the seeds individually, or one large one if you're planting them all together. The basic tools that every gardener should own include a spade, a fork, secateurs, a gardening knife, a hoe, a garden rake, a wheelbarrow and a watering can.

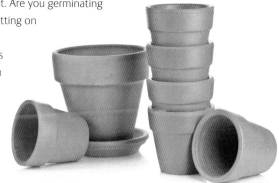

What to Consider

When you are buying tools, don't just pick up the first fork or spade you come across. There are a number of points you should consider. The first is the quality of the tools: will they last? Will they be strong enough for the tasks you need to carry out? You should also check that the tools fit you. If you are tall, make sure that you pick the right height for any tool that you will use standing up, such as a fork, hoe or rake. If they are too short to use comfortably, you could end up with backache. The same applies for people who are shorter: make sure that the length of the tool handles fit you.

If you are planting a slightly bigger eucalyptus into a larger pot you will probably only need the pot and a trowel with which to fill it with soil. The rest you can do with your hands. In order to plant a larger eucalyptus (ideally from about 0.3 m/1 ft to 1 m/3¼ ft), you will need a garden fork and/or spade, with which to dig a hole for your plant, and a hose or watering can so that you can water the eucalyptus in.

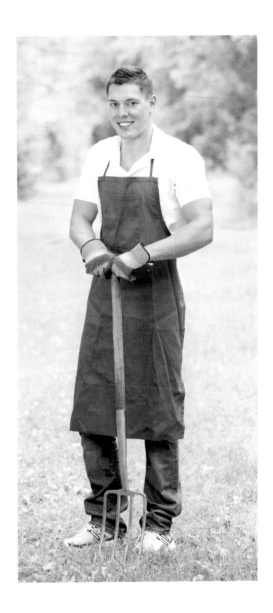

Hand Tools

A garden trowel is one of the most useful tools you can own. It is needed for lifting small amounts of compost into containers or planting spaces in your garden and can, of course, be used for additives such as grit and sand. Hand forks are also useful for a variety of tasks including tackling an area of weeds (eucalyptus plants need to grow in a weed–free area until they are established) and loosening compacted soil. The most robust hand tools are usually those made of metal, with wooden or rubber handles.

Scoops

You can usually get these useful items in metal or plastic. They can be handy for picking up compost; a large scoop can hold more compost than a trowel, and you'll be less likely to spill it. They come in a range of sizes, so you can measure out different amounts if you need to know how much fertilizer you are adding to a plant (although this is not the case for eucalyptus).

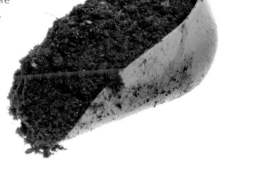

Trays

Plastic trays can be useful in many ways, such as helping to avoid waste and mess when potting and repotting. Simply put the plant and pots you're working with in the tray; any compost that spills over the edges will land in the tray, and be clean and ready to use. You can also use them to carry a number of small pots at the same time and for mixing compost with other planting material.

Cutting Tools

Secateurs are another vital part of the gardener's toolbox. All-purpose secateurs can be used on most plants grown in containers and will be useful when you come to prune the eucalyptus you have planted in pots. It's worth buying a decent pair of secateurs, if you can afford it, as this is a tool you'll use often. It may also be worth investing in a pair of florists' scissors, for more delicate jobs, such as deadheading plants and trimming herbs. They may also be handy if you need to trim small stems of eucalyptus for flower arrangements.

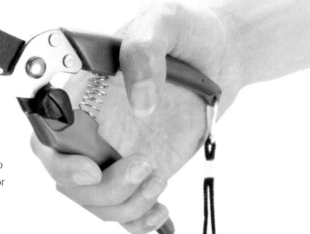

Watering Equipment

A decent watering can is
something no gardener
should be without. Choose
one that has a removable
rose, which will be crucial when
you want to get water straight
to the roots of the plant rather
than all over the flowers. A rose which
has large holes may deliver too heavy a
shower on smaller plants, so when you
are watering seedlings or bedding plants,
treat them gently and chose a rose with fine, small holes for a more delicate sprinkling.

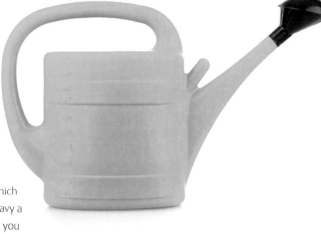

Gardening Gloves

If you belong to the school of rugged gardening you may only use these when
you're carrying out tougher jobs or tackling thorny plants. In that case, you
need a good pair of strong, protective gloves that may withstand
the onslaught from roses and brambles. However, if you
like wearing gloves for more delicate
work, too, it may be
worth investing in a
lighter pair that will
help to keep your
hands clean and to
protect you from
minor scrapes.

Choosing a Eucalyptus

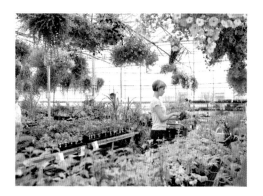

Size Matters

There are a number of factors you need to consider before deciding on the species of eucalyptus that you'd like to plant. Climate, soil type, exposure to sun and height are all important elements to consider before you make your choice. One of the main characteristics of eucalyptus trees is that they grow very tall, very quickly. Unless you have a lot of land and no close neighbours, you may want to choose a smaller–growing eucalyptus. These are often called Mallee – for instance, Plunkett Mallee (*E.curtisii*) – and branch out in a similar way to a large shrub or smallish tree. The Plunkett Mallee grows to, on average, 7 m/23 ft; the Dwarf Angophora grows to 5 m/16 ft.

Seeking Sunshine

You also need to check whether the eucalyptus you've chosen will survive in your local climatic conditions. Eucalyptus trees are native to Australia, Tasmania and a few nearby islands, so most thrive in hot temperatures. Some will cope with a degree of shade, but not all (*see* page 16). You also need to think about how cold it can be in your area, as freezing temperatures can kill the top part of the tree. The Mallee scrubs (as mentioned above) often do well on poor sandy soils, with relatively low annual rainfall such as, for instance, 350 mm/14 in. If you are unsure, ask a local eucalyptus enthusiast or garden nursery for advice on the best eucalyptus species for your area.

Location

Soil Type

The soil in which it's planted will give your eucalyptus water, nutrients and a stable base, so it's important to make sure that it's suitable for your plant. Most eucalypts prefer their soil to be well drained. Sandy soil, which is very loose, is well drained but doesn't contain many nutrients to help the plant grow. Sandy loam and loam soils have good drainage and are better at holding nutrients. Clay, on the other hand, is dense and, while it holds the nutrients that plants need, doesn't drain at all well.

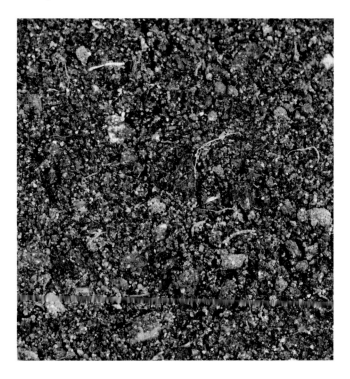

In their native Australia, plenty of species of eucalypts thrive on well-drained, shallow soil without many nutrients, so you will probably become used to seeing the warning that you should not give fertilizer to your plant (see Mulching, page 178).

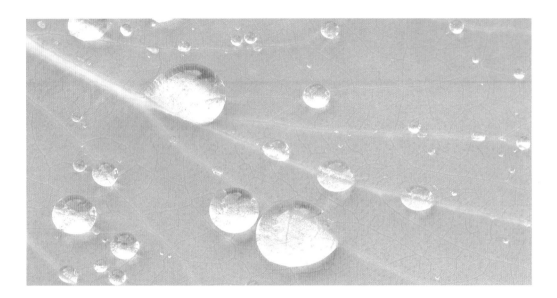

Drainage

Drainage is an important factor in choosing a location for your eucalyptus as, when first planted, they do need enough water to establish themselves. The more hardy species tend to grow naturally in areas that have around 800 mm/31 in of rain a year. More mature trees can survive a tougher drought, but they may need watering if the ground becomes very dry. If you live in an area prone to drought, choose a eucalyptus that can survive this type of weather, such as Eucalyptus cinerea (which grows to an average of 10 m/30 ft).

On the other hand, if you are planting on soil that drains poorly or tends to become waterlogged, choose a species that can survive in these wetter conditions, such as Eucalyptus neglecta (which grows to 5–10 m/15–30 ft). In Australia and Tasmania eucalypts grow in a wide range of areas, with average annual rainfall ranging from about 150 mm /6 in to more than 2,540 mm/100 in . So in terms of drought tolerance there should be a plant to suit your conditions.

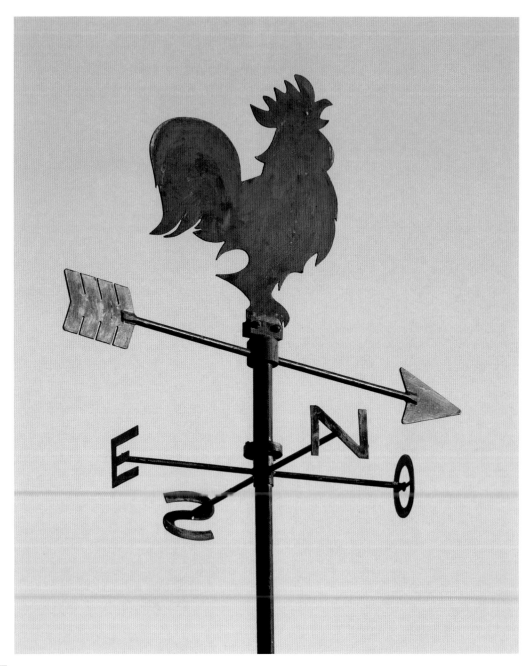

Wind Power

If you're going to be planting your eucalyptus in a cooler climate than they would enjoy in Australia, try to find a spot that, as well as having as much sunshine as possible, also provides some shelter from the wind. Not only will this protect your plant from being buffeted by cold winds, but it could also help to keep it upright.

Eucalyptus can be affected by wind rock: when the wind blows hard enough to push them partially, or totally, over. If a tree is planted when it has become root–bound (even slightly) or when it is too large, there is a tendency for the top part of the tree to grow more quickly than the roots. This can make them unstable and can mean that they may not be able to withstand the force of a strong wind.

Putting Down Roots

Eucalypts develop extensive roots. The taproot needs to go down at least six feet into the soil, as this helps to anchor the tree, while the side, or lateral, roots spread outwards from the tree by up to 30.5 m/100 ft. This helps to supply the tree with the water it needs to grow, but the roots can cause damage to buildings, pipes, etc., so you need to think carefully about where you plant your tree.

Time of Year to Plant

An important point to remember about eucalypts is that it's best to plant them as soon as possible after buying them so that they don't become root- or pot-bound. Once this has happened, they don't grow as well or as vigorously. In many parts of their native land, eucalypts can be planted at most times of year. However, if you live in a cooler climate and you're planting your tree in the ground (rather than a pot) it's better to plant in mid- to late spring, so that the plant has as much time as possible to grow before winter arrives. This is something to bear in mind before you buy a eucalyptus. And if you live in a place with hot, dry summers, be prepared to water your plant regularly to give it the best chance to grow before winter comes.

Sunny or Shady?

Eucalyptus trees are definitely sun-lovers, preferring bright sunshine to any shade. They grow best when in the sun, and the more shade they have the less well they grow, with a tendency in some to become rather 'leggy'. There are, however, some species that do well in cooler temperatures and that can manage with some shade. Eucalyptus crenulata and Eucalyptus neglecta can tolerate some shade and are probably good choices for temperate or maritime climates.

Happy Companions

When deciding where to grow your eucalypts, it might also be worth considering which other plants they should be nearby as eucalyptus can make a great companion. Eucalypts are natural insect repellants and so great for keeping those pesky pests away from your other plants. Eucalypts are particularly good at discouraging aphids and cabbage loopers, so if you are growing anything which seems to be affected by these, consider planting some eucalyptus nearby.

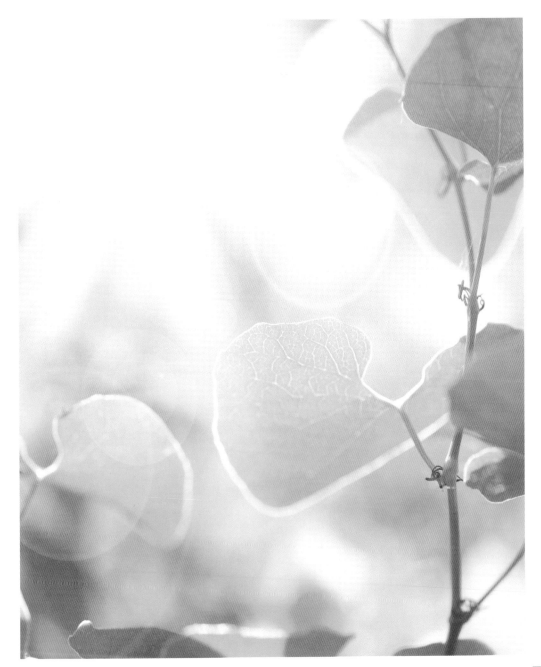

How to Grow

There is something very rewarding about growing plants, whether you have sown them as seeds or have bought them as young plants ready to move on to the next stage. Adding to the shape, smell and colour of the vegetation around you, whether it's in your garden or in your home, is a satisfying experience and helps to connect us with a slower pace of life. Even if the plant isn't native to where you live, as may be the case with eucalypts, planting and growing them is reasonably straightforward — and it can prove to be a relaxing pursuit.

Planting in Containers

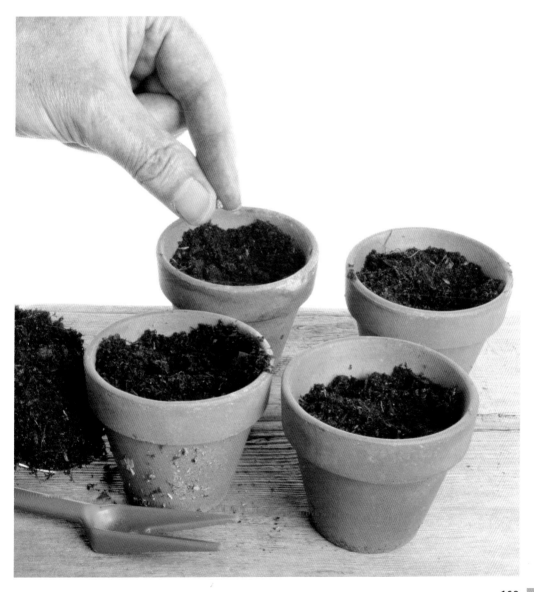

A Good Idea

Container plants have a lot to recommend them. They are portable, so you can move them around the garden and around your home, and if you move house they can come with you, which means that you don't have to leave a much-loved plant behind (eucalypts don't respond well when transplanted).

If you are certain that your plant is going to stay permanently in a pot it can make choosing a species a simpler matter. On the other hand, selecting the right plant for outdoor planting has to take into account the ultimate height and spread of the tree, as well as soil, wind and temperature.

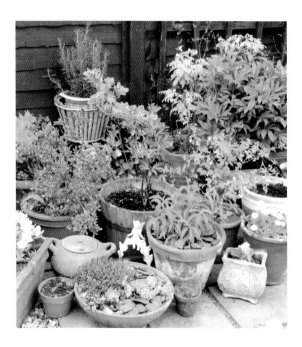

Making a Choice

Choosing a plant that you know is going to spend its life in a container is a little less complicated. You need to choose a species you like, and you need to be sure that it is healthy. One of the most important points is to check the plant's roots. Plants that have already spent too long in a pot and whose roots have become pot-bound and grow in a spiral pattern around the inside of the pot are usually regarded as being difficult to grow. Always try to start with a plant that isn't pot-bound, as you will have a better chance of successfully nurturing it.

Starting Out

When your young plant arrives, repot it into a long pot – 20–22 cm/8–9 in to allow room for the roots – using potting compost. Water the plant well and put it in a south–facing window, with bright light. This is very important if you want the plant to do well. Another point to remember is that your plant will only put on growth if the room temperature is over 8 C/46 F.

You can water your plant during the winter, but only lightly if the temperature in the room drops – just enough to keep the compost moist. Repot your plant as it grows, being very careful not to damage the roots as you do this (see page 174 for advice on how to keep your eucalyptus at a suitable size for a container plant).

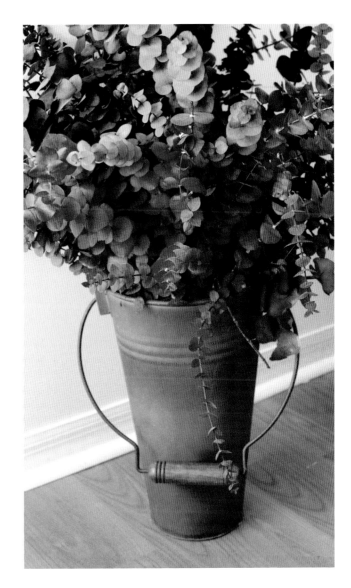

Seedlings

If you would like to grow more eucalypts from the plant you already have, the best method is to grow them from seed – a job you should do in late winter. You may have to be patient while waiting for your seeds to ripen, as they can take over a year to be ready. You'll know it's the right time to collect them when the seeds split easily. Although it may seem a little odd, for best results you should keep hardy eucalyptus seeds in your refrigerator for about two months, as this helps to encourage germination.

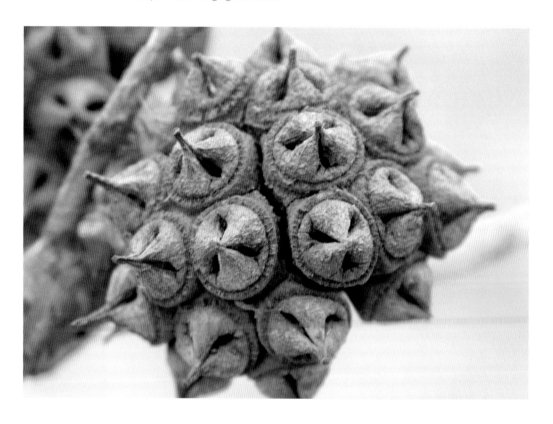

A Gentle Approach

As we have already seen, eucalypts don't do well when their roots are disturbed. In order to avoid this – and the problem of them becoming pot-bound – plant your seeds in root trainers (also known as long pots). Also use peat-free compost and provide heat from underneath the pot if possible.

Alternatively, you can sow your seeds in a tray (5–7 cm/2–3 in deep) to allow the main root room to grow. Fill the tray with peat-free compost, water it and leave to drain. Then, if you have one, put the tray in a propagator for a day or so to bring the temperature up to 15–20°C/59–68°F. Sprinkle your eucalyptus seeds onto the compost and put them back in the propagator. Make sure they don't dry out – a light spray of water on to the compost should be enough. Once your seeds have germinated (usually after one or two weeks), move them to a sunny spot.

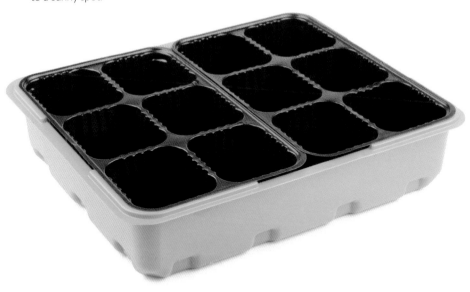

The Next Stage

When two proper leaves have grown (not the initial leaves that appear at germination), prepare the pots for the next stage. These need to be large enough for your seedlings to grow comfortably and to allow the roots to grow without being damaged. You could choose to use larger long pots or just much bigger plant pots – some gardeners use 1–gallon plant pots, which will allow the seedlings to grow until they are ready for planting outside. This means you can avoid repotting them, which brings with it the risk of damaging the roots.

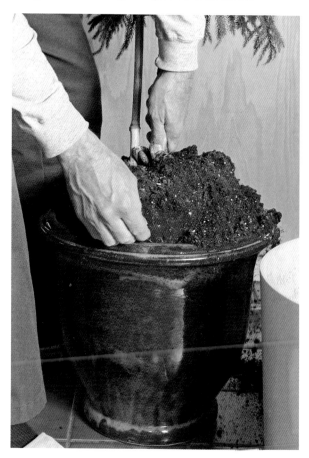

Time to Move

When you move the seedlings and young plants to repot them, hold them by their leaves and take great care not to interfere with, or damage, their roots. Ideally, in a temperate climate, you should plant the seedling out – either into pots or into the ground, depending on where you have chosen for them to grow permanently – by mid–summer or when they are over 30 cm/1 ft high.

Potting Compost

Potting compost is a vital part of any gardener's equipment, especially if you want to grow your own plants from seeds, pot young plants and repot existing plants. Most composts fall into one of two categories: those based on soil and those based on peat. Composts that are soil-based drain easily and have a fine texture. Peat-based composts are usually more fibrous.

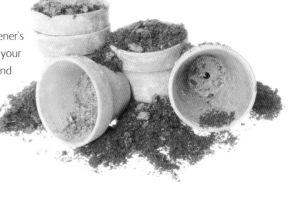

Soil-based composts are made up of a mixture of sterilized soil, also known as loam, and sand and plant nutrients. These composts have a loose, open texture but are quite heavy. Soil-less composts are often labelled as multi-purpose; they tend to be cheaper than soil-based composts and are also lighter. However, the fibrous material they contain can clump together, and this can interfere with the compost's drainage.

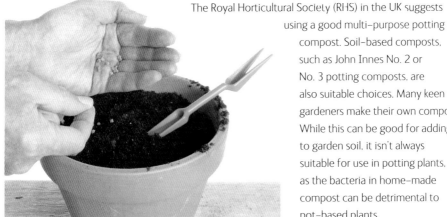

The Royal Horticultural Society (RHS) in the UK suggests using a good multi-purpose potting compost. Soil-based composts, such as John Innes No. 2 or No. 3 potting composts, are also suitable choices. Many keen gardeners make their own compost. While this can be good for adding to garden soil, it isn't always suitable for use in potting plants, as the bacteria in home-made compost can be detrimental to pot-based plants.

Planting in the Ground

First Things First

You should plant your eucalyptus in the ground as soon as possible after buying it. The first thing to do after your plant arrives home is to soak it in a bucket of water for 10–15 minutes. You should also make sure that the plant isn't top-heavy, with a root base that is smaller than its branches and leaves, and that it isn't too big. Large and top-heavy eucalypts are seen as being poor choices, as they are likely to be difficult to grow. Eucalypts do much better if they are planted when small.

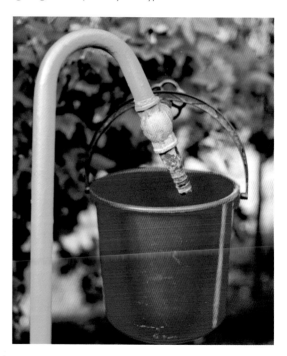

While the plant is soaking, check that the hole you have dug to plant it in is just a little larger than the plant's root ball. It isn't a good idea to include peat or other matter intended to improve the soil, as this can interfere with the movement of water around the roots; in summer it can make the effects of drought worse, and in winter it can cause heavy soils to hold more water. Also, adding manure when planting your new tree can encourage too much leafy growth, which can make the tree top-heavy and therefore more vulnerable to wind rock.

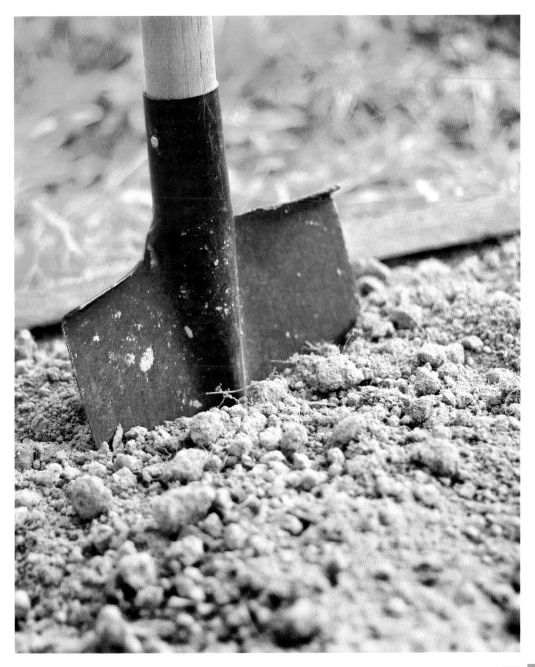

Showing Some Support

When planting your young eucalyptus outside, lower it gently into the hole you've prepared for it. Fill in, gently, around the root ball but don't cover the top level of soil already around your plant, and then water the plant in. You shouldn't need to stake young eucalypts; in fact, if the tree is allowed to grow unsupported it is more likely to develop stronger roots. The exception to this is when you are planting your tree on an exposed site, where it may be vulnerable to strong winds. In this case it can be a good idea to use a strong but short stake (at least 5 cm/2 in in diameter) and tie the plant to it at a height of 30 cm/1 ft, at most.

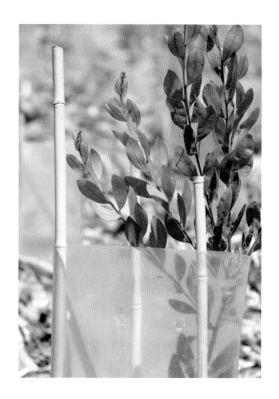

Mulching

Although eucalypts don't need much looking after once they are established, lavish a little care on them when they're young and still vulnerable. Mulching is one way in which you can do a little extra for your plant.

Mulch is a covering of either biodegradable or non-biodegradable material that is put on top of the soil in the garden around plants, or around the stems or trunks of plants in pots. A covering of mulch helps to keep moisture in the ground during the summer, to keep weeds down, to improve the texture of the soil and to protect the roots of plants from extreme heat and cold.

Mulching will help your young plant by deterring weeds and grass from growing around it and using up valuable nutrients. The mulch will also help to keep the ground moist, by slowing down water loss through evaporation. Suitable biodegradable mulching materials include wood chippings, processed bark, leaves and grass clippings. It's best not to use material that contains a lot of nitrogen, such as manure, as this can promote weed growth and can encourage the top part of the tree to grow more than the roots, thus making it unbalanced.

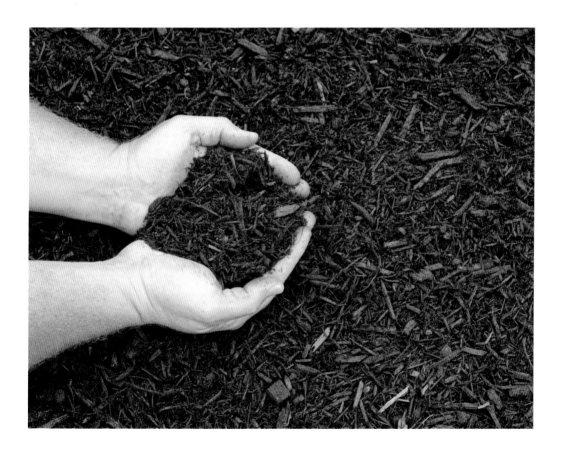

Maintenance

Planting a eucalyptus tree in your garden gives you the promise of many years – perhaps even a lifetime – of the enjoyment that comes from this species. These trees aren't fragile plants; they don't need cosseting, but it does pay to tend them during the first few years. Once they are well established and have put down strong roots, you will be able to enjoy them all year round. And knowing what to watch out for means that if a problem does arise, you'll know how to deal with it.

Basic Care

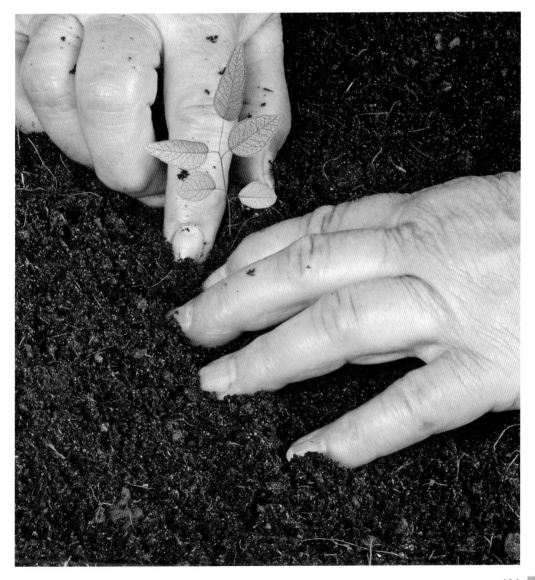

Watering and Feeding

It is important to make sure that your eucalyptus is well watered before you plant it. And you must carry on watering it thoroughly, possibly as often as every day, if it is in very porous soil. Your newly planted tree will be vulnerable for a while, until it is well established, so don't let it dry out. A light sprinkling can cause shallow rooting, so it's better to soak the area with a couple of watering canfuls.

If you live in an area with frequent rain you may not need to water at all, but keep an eye on the situation if you want your tree to stay healthy. Mulching (see page 178) can help to prevent moisture loss. Once your tree is well established it shouldn't really need watering, except in particularly dry periods. As for feeding, the general advice is not to feed ground-planted eucalypts, as they don't need it.

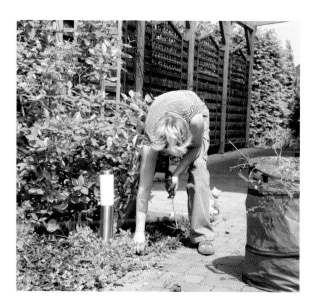

Weeding

Weeding around the base of your tree is also important, because weeds and grass will compete with the eucalyptus for moisture and nutrients. Ideally, you should have an area of at least 60 cm/2 ft radius that is weed- and grass-free; achieving this for the first two years will help your tree grow well. Mulching can help with this or you can use woven landscape fabric, which you can camouflage with bark, gravel, etc.

Pruning

Eucalypts are such fast-growing and tall trees that they can quickly become too big for all but the very largest gardens. However, there are a number of ways, such as coppicing or pruning that can help you enjoy a eucalyptus in your garden without the tree towering over the neighbourhood. Coppicing can create a multi-stemmed bush rather than a single-stemmed tree and it should be carried out in late winter to early spring (February to March in the UK, but this could be different in other countries), before the trees start their spring/summer growth.

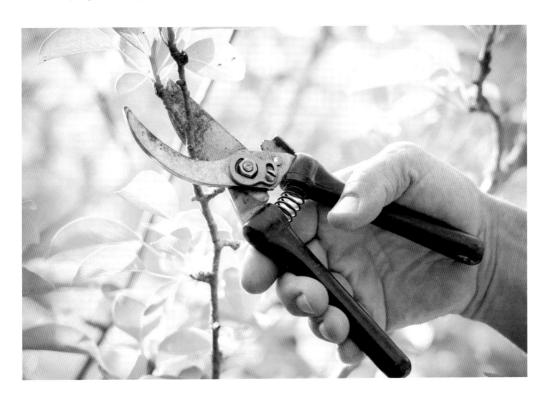

You can prune eucalypts so they remain a standard tree height (1–2 m/3¼–6½ ft trunk) by following these instructions:

In the first year you should cut off all the side branches on the bottom third of the tree and cut the side shoots on the middle third to half their length. In year two remove the shoots you cut in half the previous year. Then cut the side shoots on what is now the middle third of the tree to half their length. Finally, cut off the branches that cross over each other in the upper section of the tree. Repeat the process you carried out in year two also in year three.

In the years that follow you can control growth and neaten the tree by removing side branches from the trunk, so that the tree stays at the height you want it to be. Carry on taking off diseased, dead and straggly branches from the upper levels.

Coppicing

Coppicing is a good approach to take if you want your eucalyptus to grow as a multi-stemmed bush and to provide foliage for floral arrangements. Eucalyptus leaves are popular in many kinds of floral displays, because of their interesting shapes and delicate colours. A method often used for coppicing is to leave the eucalyptus growing in the ground for two or three years and then to cut it down to just one or two feet from the ground. By the following year branches will have grown out of the remaining trunk, both from the cut area and below ground level. Choose three or four of the best branches to keep and cut the others off at the base.

From the following year onwards, trim off the unsuitable side shoots – those that hang too low, for instance, or cross over and rub on each other. You should also cut off any new side stems growing from the original trunk. You should now have a plant that will carry on developing as a multi-stemmed bush, of a manageable height, and it should now be a simple task to harvest the best stems for flower arrangements.

CAUTION: Pruning and coppicing may involve working with heavy, sharp tools, and climbing. Take great care when carrying out this work. Always wear safety equipment – goggles, gloves and protective clothing – and have someone with you while you work, in case of emergency. If the task is more than you can safely cope with, employ a professional arborist or tree surgeon to do the work.

Pollarding

Pollarding is another approach that can restrict the growth of eucalypts once they have reached your preferred height. However, this is a more complicated job, which requires a head for heights, so is really best left to a professional such as an arborist (or tree surgeon).

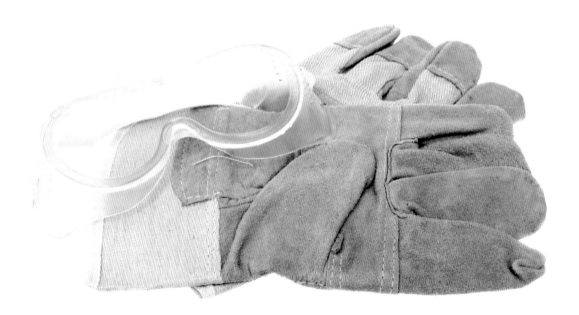

Pests

Longhorned Borers

Eucalypts are quite hardy plants, but they can still be affected by pests, including one that can cause fatal damage to the tree. Eucalyptus longhorned borers lay their eggs in the bark of eucalyptus trees. After they have hatched, the larvae bore their way into the inner bark and, once there, they feed on a thin layer of tissue on the bark's inner surface, sometimes creating chambers several feet long. Once the feeding period is over, the larvae pupate in the chambers they have created and then emerge as adult beetles, ready to lay their own eggs.

These beetles usually target trees that are under stress – often because of drought or lack of nutrients. You can help to keep them at bay by making sure your eucalyptus has enough water and by removing dead and dying branches from the tree and the area near it.

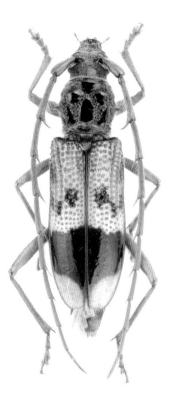

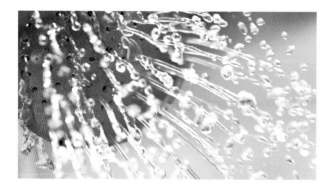

Red Gum Lerp Psyllid

Psyllids are probably one of the most damaging pests to eucalypts and something you don't want to find on your tree. The adult eucalyptus red gum lerp psyllids are about 3 cm/⅛ in long and range in colour from light green to brownish, with orange and yellow blotches. The females lay eggs on young leaves and shoots, and the nymphs emerge several weeks to several months later, depending on the temperature. The nymphs create a white, domed cover or 'lerp' over themselves out of solidified honeydew (which they secrete) and wax.

The red gum, also known as eucalyptus camaldulensis, is just one of the 26 varieties of eucalyptus that is affected by the red gum lerp psyllid, but it's the one that is hit the hardest. The damage caused by the psyllids results in the tree losing its leaves and, if the problem continues, becoming stressed. In this condition they can become more vulnerable to other pests. In the worst cases the trees can die.

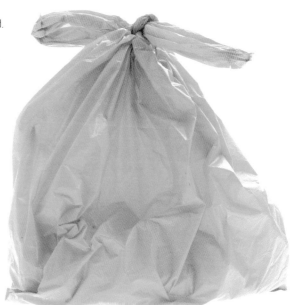

In order to combat a psyllid infestation, encourage their natural enemies, such as pirate bugs and parasitic wasps (you will have to check to see if these are local to your area). You can also put sticky traps on the branches to capture the adults and also remove branches that are badly affected. Put these branches into plastic bags when you dispose of them to reduce the risk of contaminating other trees in the area.

Gall Wasps

The eucalyptus gall wasp is a tiny black insect. The adults are about 1 mm long and appear in late May to June. The adult females lay their eggs on young eucalyptus leaves in early summer. The larvae grow inside the leaves, and raised galls (bumps) develop around them, but don't become really obvious until almost a year later, when the larvae have grown. The galls grow on either side of the leaves and are about 1 mm in diameter. A heavy infestation of gall wasps spoils the appearance of the older leaves in springtime and can cause a heavier than expected leaf fall.

If the affected eucalyptus is small enough for you to be able to reach all the branches, you can spray it with a systemic insecticide (such as thiacloprid or acetamiprid) in late spring/early summer, but these substances are not a popular choice for many people. You also have to consider the effect they may have on the other insects and plants in your and neighbouring gardens. You can also gather up and destroy the affected leaves when they fall in the spring, which will stop some of the gall wasps reaching maturity.

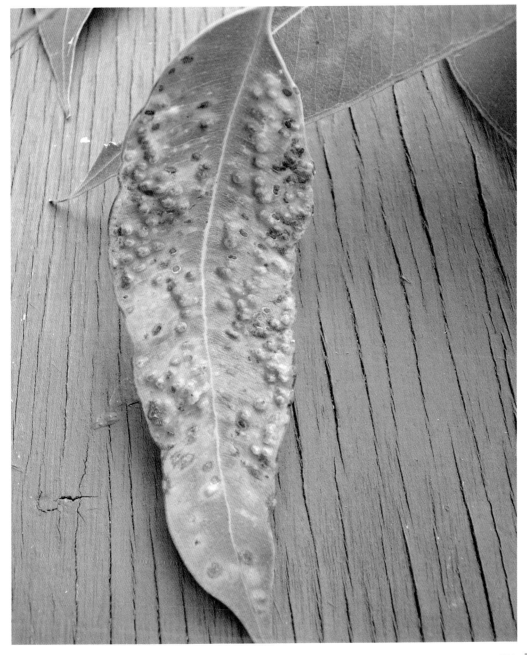

Index

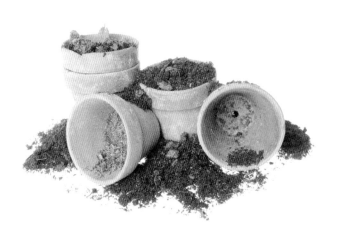